Contents

Acknowledgments

Many thanks to everyone who has contributed
to the making of this book.

Special thanks to Mum and Dad for
constant love and support.

For more information about other books by the same author visit
www.healingbooks.co.uk

Introduction

In recent years hand reflexology has become better known and more widely used than ever before. One of the obvious benefits is the ease of access to the hands and no one minds having their hands massaged; sometimes foot reflexology can be inconvenient and might feel too "invasive" for some people. It is also very easy to treat yourself with hand reflexology but not so easy to reach your own feet! Bearing this in mind and the fact that the results can be at least as successful as foot reflexology, this simple but powerful healing technique seems set to stay.

I became interested in reflexology after suffering from chronic fatigue syndrome for a few years. A friend told me about it so I looked in a local telephone directory and found a qualified therapist. The first treatment was so relaxing that I fell asleep and there was a definite improvement in my mental outlook after the second and third treatments. Each time I went for a treatment I also felt that some kind of natural healing process was being triggered or stimulated within my body. At the same time I became aware of two other types of natural healing therapies, Reiki and the Bach Flower Remedies. Through combining these three therapies my health improved and I was able to lead a normal life again. I was so taken with the gentle power of reflexology that I decided to train to become a qualified practitioner. During the training we were taught hand and foot reflexology, although the main emphasis was on the latter. It was not until I began to practice after qualifying that I realized how special hand reflexology can be.

Hand reflexology can work on many levels; you can just regard it as a physical therapy for relaxing the mind and stimulating the natural healing process within the body. However, the power of hand reflexology is often underestimated, sometimes just holding someone's hand when they are in distress can be very healing. It would not have the same effect if you held someone's foot when they were upset! When you hold someone's hand it is almost as if you are holding their heart. If someone allows you to hold their hand it is as if they are opening their heart to you and in this sense hand reflexology can be more powerful than foot reflexology.

All deep, long-lasting healing comes from healing the heart. What is the "heart"? Thoughts and feelings are part of the mind and the heart is a special part of the mind, the center of the mind, the center of our being. Illness can often result from having and holding negative thoughts and feelings and healing can often result from transforming our negative minds into positive minds. By healing the heart we are going to the heart of the problem, where all thoughts and feelings come from. To have a healthy heart means to have a sense of inner peace, to be at peace with ourselves and the world around us. If we have inner peace ourselves we can give it to others and hand reflexology is a great way to pass this on. We are influenced greatly by the people we spend time with and as therapists we are allowed into the close personal space of another person, because of this we can influence them greatly in obvious and more subtle ways. Spending time with a therapist who has a deep sense of inner peace, apart from their physical skill, can be a large part of the healing process. So if you want to become a successful healer you need to learn the physical skills required but you also need to learn how to heal your own heart, then you can help others do the same. If you have a sense of inner peace, contentment, and happiness there is not much more that you need in life. Taking the time to develop these inner qualities is really the solution to so many of the problems we experience in daily life. Everyone is looking for happiness; all the decisions and choices we make come from this one wish. We choose our career, partner, house, etc. because they make us feel good in some way. Even when we choose a particular brand of biscuits we choose one that we like, we never choose to suffer. Yet happiness is just a state of mind.

A happy mind means a happy life; even if you experience health, relationship, or financial problems if you can keep a happy mind you will be happy! This is easier said than done but it can be done if you train your mind wisely and patiently over months and years. This training is one of the main aspects of the Buddhist path but you do not have to be Buddhist to benefit from these teachings and they can be very valuable for a healer/therapist to learn. Often physical healing comes much more swiftly to someone with a happy and peaceful outlook, and it is obvious that strong negative states of mind like depression and grief have an adverse effect on the body. So, in conclusion, if you learn the techniques in this book you will become a good healer but if you also learn to heal your heart you will become a special type of healer, the type of healer that the world really needs. For this reason I have included some information on the Buddhist path, which may give you some helpful ideas and start you in the right direction, but if you want to take this further the best way is to find a qualified teacher (see Appendix 1).

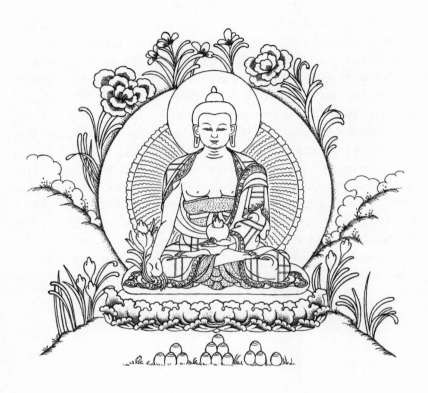

1

History
of reflexology

The actual origins of reflexology are lost in the past; we do not know exactly when or where it began. We know that some form of this therapy was performed in ancient China, India, and Egypt but we do not know exactly how far back they date. Our modern therapy developed without the knowledge of these systems, which would seem to suggest that it is a valid form of healing born from experience and success, becoming well established in four very different cultures. The Chinese have had an accurate and detailed understanding of the human body for thousands of years, and reflexology became a part of their system of medicine because it was a very effective way of rebalancing the internal energy system of the body. It was found that many of the meridians (life force energy pathways) run through the feet and hands, so a system of massage developed from this knowledge. Here is a brief explanation of the Chinese system of medicine; a more detailed explanation is given later:

> Traditional Chinese medicine is a holistic system of healing which has diagnosed, treated, and prevented illness for at least 3000 years.
>
> Based on the principles of internal balance and harmony, this highly refined and complex discipline works to regenerate the

body's organs and systems ... Each human is viewed as a mini-ecosystem that shares common traits with the earth on which we live.

The Chinese have a concept of vital energy known as chi or qi (pronounced chee), which is the basis of all life. In the body, chi is transported via the 12 major energetic pathways known as meridians. Although these meridians cannot be seen with the naked eye, modern science has proven their existence through electronic detection. Each meridian connects to one of the major organs, and chi is said to power the organ, enabling effective functioning. For example, the path of the heart meridian travels from the heart, to the armpit, and down the inside of the arm to the little finger. This explains why some individuals with heart conditions will express a tingling feeling running down the arm and into the fingers. Chi is regulated by the interdependent forces of yin and yang.

The Chinese symbol for yin literally means "the dark side of the mountain", and represents the qualities of cold, still, dark, below, weakness, and void. The Chinese symbol for yang translates to "the sunny side of the mountain", and therefore represents the opposite qualities of yin: heat, activity, light, above strength, and solidity. A person's constitution, or the nature of the disease, is determined by the aspects of yin and yang. Harmony and balance of this union yields a healthy state, whereas excess or deficiency of either yin or yang is thought to lead to illness.

Source: www.aworldofchinesemedicine.com

The modern school

Modern reflexology developed separately from any influence of Chinese medicine or acupuncture. However, reflexologists today take a great interest in this field of knowledge and apply it to their practice. Although you do not need such knowledge to become an accomplished reflexologist, an awareness of meridian theory is very useful and an understanding of life force energy can greatly improve your understanding of the healing process.

The modern system began with the development of zone

therapy by a man called Dr. Fitzgerald. Born and brought up in Connecticut, USA, Fitzgerald qualified as a doctor and studied with interest the techniques of Dr. H Bressler from Vienna who was researching techniques for treating certain conditions with pressure points.

Dr. Fitzgerald began his own research in to this area while working as the head physician at the Hartford Ear, Nose, and Throat Hospital in Connecticut. The first thing that he discovered was that if constant pressure was applied to the fingers it would create an anesthetic effect in the hand, arm, shoulder, neck, and face on the same side of the body. With this anesthetic effect he was even able to carry out minor surgery to the numbed areas. He further discovered that the body could be divided into 10 vertical zones running from head to toe and corresponding to the 10 fingers and toes, so that pressure applied to certain fingers would have an effect on parts of the body contained within the corresponding zones.

This extract from the book *Zone Therapy* by Dr. Fitzgerald and Dr. Bowers, published in 1917, explains how Dr. Fitzgerald discovered and developed his ideas:

> I accidentally discovered that pressure with a cotton tipped probe on the mucocutaneous margin of the nose gave an anaesthetic result as though a cocaine solution had been applied. I further found that there were many spots in the nose, mouth, throat, and on both surfaces of the tongue which, when pressed firmly, deadened definite areas of sensation. Also, that pressures exerted over any body eminence, on the hands, feet or over the joints, produced the same characteristic results in pain relief. I found also that when pain was relieved, the condition that produced the pain was most generally relieved. This led to my "mapping out" these various areas and their associated connections, and also to noting the conditions influenced through them. This science I have named zone therapy.

One of Dr. Fitzgerald's colleagues wrote an article entitled, "To Stop That Toothache Squeeze Your Toe!" which was published in 1915. This caused great interest at the time and many people became interested in zone therapy. Dr. Fitzgerald and his colleagues often experienced skepticism from their medical colleagues and sometimes, to prove their theories, if the skeptic was brave enough, they would anesthetize an area of their face by applying pressure to the relevant finger and then push a pin into the skin. This would quickly convert the skeptic to a believer!

Once Dr. Fitzgerald was asked, at a dinner party, what zone therapy could do for one of the guests present who was a professional singer. The upper register of her voice had gone flat and this was causing her great concern. She had already consulted medical specialists who could not help her. Dr. Fitzgerald looked at her throat and then to the amusement of the other guests he asked to look at the singer's hands and feet. After a short examination he told her that her problem was simply caused by the formation of a callus on her right big toe! This caused much amusement but the doctor simply smiled and applied pressure to the callused area for a few minutes. The doctor asked her to try the upper register of her voice; not only was she able to easily reach the notes she had been "missing" but she was able to reach two tones higher than she had ever done before!

Unfortunately zone therapy was not developed any further at that time, possibly because much of what was discovered was not regarded with much respect or interest by the medical profession. One doctor who did have a high regard for Fitzgerald's work was Dr. Joseph Shelby Riley. Dr. Riley and his wife Elizabeth were taught zone therapy by Dr. Fitzgerald and applied it in their medical practice for many years. It was Riley who made the first detailed drawings and diagrams of the reflex points located on the feet. He wrote four books covering all aspects of zone therapy.

A lady called Eunice Ingham was one of Dr. Riley's assistants and she is now widely regarded as the mother of modern reflexology. Eunice spent many years researching and developing techniques, which transformed the fairly basic and unrefined methods of zone therapy into the technically detailed healing practice we know today.

She was particularly enthusiastic about sharing her knowledge with non-medical or lay practitioners in the hope that many people would learn her techniques and practice on friends and family. She was not bothered about recognition from the medical profession as she had seen the way they had reacted to zone therapy. She knew that the methods she was developing were effective for healing all manner of conditions and she simply wanted many people to benefit from this knowledge.

Eunice discovered that the whole body could be mapped out through the reflexes on the feet, as if the feet were a mirror of the whole body. As the excellent results of her work continued word spread and people from miles around came to see her and receive treatments. Eunice's nephew, Dwight Byers, received many treatments for his asthma and hay fever and his aunt talked to him during those treatments about her work and how her research was developing. Today Dwight runs the International Institute of Reflexology.

Eunice Ingham also wrote two books, which are seminal texts for all those interested in practicing reflexology. They are *Stories The Feet Can Tell* (1938) and *Stories The Feet Have Told* (1963). If Eunice could now be aware of the extent to which her work has benefited others and has been embraced by millions of people worldwide, she would be very pleased.

Reflexology has not replaced zone therapy, indeed many reflexologists use it as a useful aid to the healing process and the client or patient can easily be taught to use this therapy during the time between regular reflexology treatments. Also, many reflexologists combine other therapies with their practice, like Reiki, Aromatherapy, Bach Flower Remedies, etc. These are all excellent and complementary additions to the healing program, which all modern therapists should seriously consider using.

The future of reflexology

Many reflexologists also consider it important to have a knowledge of Chinese meridian theory and some believe that the explanations this gives for how foot or hand massage stimulates healing are more accurate than that provided by zone therapy. In fact, we could say that the knowledge we have gained from meridian theory has taken reflexology forward since the discoveries of Dr. Fitzgerald and Eunice Ingham. Meridian theory is quite an in-depth subject and principally derived from what we know about acupuncture and Chinese medicine. For the moment though, it is interesting to note that reflexology is really nothing new! Many ancient civilizations were far more medically advanced than our own. They understood the subtle energies of the body and the implications that mental and emotional well-being have on physical health and they developed their healing techniques accordingly. We have lost much of this precious wisdom and modern medicine, although very valuable, sometimes blindly pursues healing from a purely physical standpoint. Most of us need to see physical evidence of anything before we believe that the "unseen" might exist. We are afraid to trust our other senses, especially the subtle ones like intuition and inner wisdom. However, gradually some people are beginning to open their eyes and consider the possibilities that there may be ways to health and happiness, other than purely conventional medicine and materialism.

There is no doubt that reflexology, like other complementary therapies, will not stand still. New developments will come and should be embraced, once tried and tested. A good therapist should always be open to new ideas, although cautious of so-called miracle cures. There is a vast amount of information about reflexology now available, much of which is published on the Internet, although to become a competent practitioner you do not have to know the ins and outs of all the theories and new developments especially if you only intend to practice on friends and family. There is much to be said for just buying and studying a few well-chosen books and practice, practice, practice!

2

How does
reflexology work?

Many reflexologists believe that the feet and hands are linked to various parts of the body by a countless number of nerve connections. It is thought that the various nerve endings in the feet and hands correspond to the "zones" of the body as explained in zone theory. It is also thought that the nerve endings correspond to the map of the human physiology. If we look at the soles of the left and right foot they appear to form the general shape of the human body with the big toes relating to the head and neck of the torso, the base of the little toes as the left and right shoulder, each instep as the left and right side of the spine and so on. A similar view can be developed for the hands, with the spine running up the inside and the thumbs being the neck and head.

However, there is no definite evidence that this is a conclusive, accurate, and definitive theory. In fact the number and complexity of nerve endings make it almost impossible to identify clearly which areas affect different parts of the body. Because the nervous system is so extensive and covers the whole body, creating pleasure or pain in just one small area has a dramatic effect on the whole. However, despite this there is so much evidence that practicing reflexology rather than simple foot or hand massage has a very beneficial effect on health that we have to admit that massaging and stimulating the feet or hands in a specific way has a more direct and positive effect on the body and mind.

An alternative theory explains reflexology through the principals of Chinese medicine. This stipulates that there are within the body a number of invisible energy pathways or meridians that carry life force energy or chi. It is said that when these pathways become blocked, perhaps due to stress, then illness can result. Sometimes acupuncture or acupressure is used to release these blockages and stimulate a free flow of healthy life force energy. As most of the major energy pathways end or begin in the feet or hands, reflexology will naturally stimulate them in some way. However, even a full reflexology treatment would not stimulate or treat all of the meridians, as they do not all end in the feet or hands and there are many minor or tributary pathways as well as the main ones. This is why acupuncture or acupressure is performed all over the body. Acupuncture is many thousands of years old so if it were most effective by treating only the feet or hands this would have been noticed by now!

The nervous system is the link between the mind and the body. We also know that the subtle internal energies, or "winds" as they are known in Buddhist philosophy, govern our mental and physical health. When we are carrying and naturally generating strong, clear, and well-balanced subtle internal winds then our physical and mental health is good. To understand these ideas it will be helpful to gain a basic understanding of what "energy" is and why it is so important and vital to life. We could say that Life Force Energy is the subtle foundation of all life, a sort of subtle "cosmic soup" that supports, nourishes, and sustains the cycle of birth, life, and death of all forms of life.

Physical matter is made up of differing frequencies of energy. Solid objects are made up of energy vibrating at a very low or slow frequency. Less solid objects like water, air, and life force energy are vibrating incredibly fast. We also know that within the molecules and atoms of matter there is proportionately more "space" than between the planets in our universe! So all is not as it seems and appearances are deceptive.

Buddhism, Vedic Science, and other similar eastern philosophies understand the concept of energy much better than we do. They also incorporate this knowledge into their religions in a way that explains the mystical and spiritual experiences that many devoted practitioners have. In these societies science, religion, and art are not separated but seen simply as branches of the same tree of life. One aspect of the eastern understanding of God is as a Universal Life Force Energy. That is, the one true source of all life. All the energy that breathes life into plants, trees, animals, humans, planets, stars, and universes comes from this one source. It is this source of life that we need to make contact with if we want to maintain or recreate good physical, mental, and spiritual health. When we are in touch with this energy through prayer, meditation, taking a walk in the countryside, or receiving healing we feel less "separate" and increasingly "whole" within ourselves and within the "whole" of creation. We experience a sense of unity, we become more aware of our place or role in the great scheme of things, and at the same time we feel supported, safe, open, and confident in our abilities to be all that we are, without doubt or apology. We can say that these spiritual or personal experiences are the "Essence" of healing and they are a pleasant byproduct of many complementary therapies.

There are two main types of Life Force Energy: Internal and External. Internal Life Force Energy is the subtle energy that exists within the body and mind of all living beings. External Life Force Energy exists within plants, flowers, trees, rocks, minerals, crystals and this energy is often harnessed for healing purposes as in the Bach Flower Remedies, Crystal Healing, Flower Essences, Homeopathic and Herbal Remedies. Even just a walk in the countryside or by the sea can have a calming and healing effect on us. There is so much pure External Life Force Energy available in these places that it "lifts" our own internal energies and this has a corresponding effect on our body and mind. Conversely, if we spend too much time in built-up areas or stressful environments where these natural energies are restricted it may adversely affect our health if we are unable to transform or "rise above" these situations. As mentioned, Internal Life Force Energy runs through subtle channels or meridians in the human body and when these are blocked or imbalanced, due to stress for example, illness can result. Most complementary therapies seek to help the body and mind rebalance and cleanse these internal energies, thereby promoting health and well-being, and this is also the way reflexology works as a healing technique.

When our Internal Life Force Energy system is blocked, sluggish, or imbalanced, regular reflexology has the effect of naturally and effortlessly dissolving and raising the quality of that energy to the healthiest level that our body, mind, and environment will allow. A reflexology treatment also has the effect of opening our energy system to again receive a well-balanced flow of Universal Life Force Energy that is often cut off or restricted by illness. Although, perhaps more accurately, we could say that being cut off from this life force is the cause of much illness.

If you are treating others it is helpful to investigate why the patient became distant from their natural relationship with the Universal Life Force and how they can work to maintain a healthy relationship with it in the future. For some this may involve a personal spiritual revolution by rediscovering their own or a new religion or perhaps looking into such practices as meditation, yoga, or Tai Chi, etc. But one does not have to get "religious" to develop this special inner relationship with life. Babies are not religious but they definitely carry a particular pure energy that comes from somewhere special! It is interesting to note that many well-known and respected spiritual teachers, healers, and saints carry a similar energy!

Inner and outer harmony

When Internal and External Life Force Energy are in harmony, posses the same level of purity, and exist on the same wavelength or frequency and within the same realm of existence they are very similar energies. The only difference is that Internal Life Force Energy has consciousness or "mind" and cannot exist separately from it. Due to the close relationship between consciousness and Internal Life Force Energy it is easy to believe that the sense of closeness or companionship we feel toward trees, crystals, the Earth, or other sources of External Life Force Energy is because they possess a personal character or mind. External Life Force Energy, like that within trees, crystals, and the Earth does not possess consciousness or mind. However, this does not make them any less special or sacred "living" objects. So our internal energies and our mind are inseparable, they exist almost as one and have a very intimate dependent relationship. In fact, although we do not generally notice it our thoughts and feelings "ride" on our internal energies. If we carry positive Internal Life Force Energy of a good quality, perhaps because it is enhanced with Reiki, it is easier for us to develop positive states of mind and we generally attract positive life experiences and deal with problems more easily. Likewise, if we consciously try to develop positive states of mind, like confidence, kindness, and wisdom, this will raise the quality of our internal energies and in turn improve our health and many other aspects of our lives.

So, in conclusion, perhaps we can say that the practice of reflexology stimulates or relaxes the nervous system, and this in turn affects the mind and our internal energy system at the same time, as they are inseparable. As will be explained in more detail later, if we possess the potential to get well then simply by treating, stimulating, relaxing, or "massaging" the mind and internal energy system through the nervous system we will naturally move toward good health. Our bodies tend to do this anyway given the right conditions. What we are doing in reflexology and other therapies is simply encouraging this process and creating the inner peace, "space," and other conditions conducive to healing.

Much of the success of reflexology is simply due to the deep physical and mental relaxation created by a reflexology treatment, as this is one of the major conditions required for us to regain our own inner healing abilities. There are many other obvious conditions like good diet, regular light exercise, social and environmental circumstances, mental attitude, etc. However, there are times when good health is not so easily restored or maintained, even when all the obvious conditions for good health are present. Then we need to look for deeper solutions and these will be examined later in a chapter on the cause and cure of disease. However, generally speaking we can see that with a good motivation reflexology can greatly assist us in improving our own and others' quality of life, helping us become more whole and healthy beings on all levels, and this in turn naturally benefits those around us and the friends and relatives of those we treat. When we help one person we are indirectly helping all those with whom our patient has a relationship.

Also, as mentioned we need to encourage the people we treat to keep a happy mind, whatever their level of health. This is one of the major conditions required for good health to return but more importantly our mind is the one thing we can control if we learn how to. We have a certain amount of control over our health but ultimately we will all become sick and have to face the process of dying and leaving behind all that we love and have worked for. If we can learn throughout our life to keep a peaceful, happy mind whatever happens and to practice contentment and patience when things go wrong, we will be good role models for others and we will leave this world with a strong and healthy mind, which can only be a cause of happiness in the future.

3

Hand reflexology techniques

Examine the hands

Before you begin to treat a new patient it is good practice to check the hands thoroughly for any medical conditions and ask the patient if they have any joint problems. You can makes notes about what you find on a case study sheet and it is useful to tell the patient what you are doing as you inspect each hand. If you find any infections, cuts, or warts just avoid that area or wear medical grade rubber gloves.

Some problems like arthritis will mean you will have to be especially gentle and careful not to cause discomfort during the treatment. It is most important that the patient's treatment is comfortable and relaxing. They will not be able to relax if they expect pain, so reassure such clients that you will be gentle and ask them to let you know if and where there is any discomfort. You can make notes about such cases to remind you for future treatments.

If you are satisfied with the inspection the next step is to loosen and relax the hands with a few simple stretching and rotating exercises. This also helps the client to relax and gain confidence in you as a therapist before the treatment begins properly. These simple exercises are given at the beginning of the next chapter.

Treatment techniques

The techniques that we use during a reflexology treatment cannot be learned quickly. It really takes years to master them until they become second nature. You can best appreciate this by receiving a treatment from a newly qualified reflexologist and from someone who has been practicing for many years – there is a big difference.

However, reflexology is such an effective and powerful form of therapy that even in the hands of complete beginners remarkable and lasting healings can take place in just a short time. So you should not be afraid to expect success and good results right from the word go. If you take your time and do not try to rush to learn all there is to know, even your very first treatment will be effective.

You should take time to learn and practice the basics. If you have a friend or partner who is a willing patient you should take advantage of this as often as possible and practice all the techniques you are learning whenever you can. Initially you may feel more comfortable practicing the basic hand techniques on your own hands. This is useful as they are always available and you will immediately gain experience of how the techniques feel to the patient. You will also learn how much pressure to apply, which is important for the patients' comfort and saves the therapist's muscles from over straining.

Supporting the hand

The usual support hold is used throughout the treatment. While one hand is working a particular set of reflexes the other is always employed to support the hand. The idea is to prevent the patient's hand from moving around too much. The patient's comfort is always of paramount importance so never grip tightly, just use one hand like a plate to take the full weight of the patient's hand and forearm.

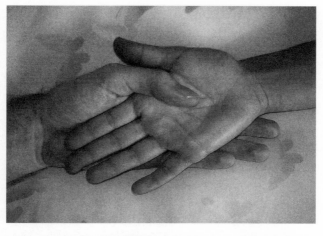

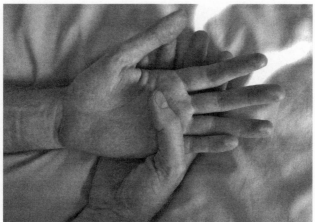

Figures 1a and 1b   Supporting the hand

Other support grips can be used when treating the side of the hands to stop the patient's hand moving away from you. Whichever side you are treating your other hand should assist by keeping the patient's hand from moving away. When you are treating yourself you can just place the hand you are working on on your knee or on a low tabletop or on a cushion, again the main criterion is to be comfortable, for the resting hand to be as relaxed as possible and for it not to move about too much.

Finger and thumb walking techniques

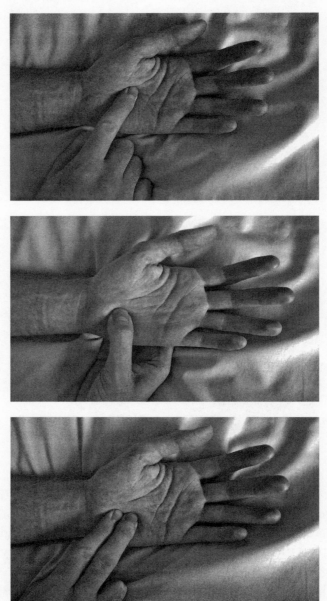

Figures 2a, 2b, and 2c   Massage techniques

These are the most used and most important techniques to learn and are used throughout the treatment. They are not difficult to master with a little practice and the best place to practice at first is simply on your own hands. This enables you to feel how much pressure you are applying. To begin, support the back of one hand with the fingers of the other or rest one hand on a cushion as shown in the figures. Then gently press the thumb or the first finger into the palm, release the pressure slowly while at the same time sliding the thumb forward slightly, just a few millimeters, then apply gentle pressure again, release, and move forward. The main point is that there should be no gaps or space between the pressure points so that not even the smallest area of skin is missed. The action should be repeated constantly while trying to move in a straight line across the palm. The whole movement is a sort of rhythmic nibbling action. You can practice all over the hands and fingers and then swap hands and practice with the other thumb. If you are right handed you will probably find it easier to use your right thumb but with practice you will be able to use both as easily; this is important as both hands are used equally during a full treatment.

The same nibbling massage action is used with the fingers. You will need to practice with the index finger on its own, the index and second finger together, and all the fingers together. This can be done on the hands or the forearms.

Some reflexologists like to combine the finger and thumb movements with a small rotating motion so that as pressure is applied you move the thumb in a tiny circular motion, usually clockwise. This is repeated with every move forward. You might like this technique and find it simple to use and it can be very effective. However, if you find it difficult just use the normal technique to begin with, and you can always come back to this later. During a treatment you could use both techniques as and when you feel it is right. Getting feedback from the patient is a helpful indicator.

Finger and thumb massage

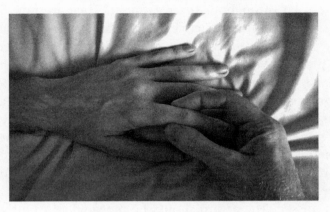

Figure 3   Finger technique

The above diagram shows the index finger being used to massage the sides of the fingers whilst the thumb supports the opposite side of the finger and the other hand is employed in the normal support grip. You can practice this technique on the fingers by supporting one side of the finger with the thumb while simply rubbing the index finger backwards and forwards in the area to be massaged. Some reflexologists use an additional circular motion so you can try this if it feels right. There is some flexibility in the techniques used in reflexology so as long as you learn the basics and do not stray too far from the orthodox treatment sequence you can apply your own experience and creativity to improve the techniques as many reflexologists have done.

Pressure technique and knuckle press/massage

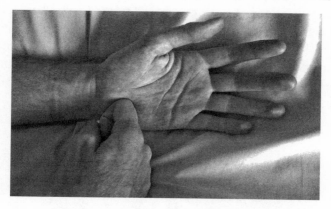

Figure 4   Knuckle technique

With this technique one or two knuckles can be gently pressed in and dragged or pressed in and gently rotated, moved slightly, and pressed and rotated again, and so on. Alternatively a kneading action can be used as though you were kneading bread. You can work from left to right or top to bottom as long as the whole of the reflex area is covered. This technique is mainly used for areas where the skin is thick or tough, for example around the base of the hands.

Pressure point hold (knuckle or thumb)

Some reflexologists find that some areas of the hands respond well to a simple pressure hold. A need for this might be indicated by skin that seems limp, puffy, or lacking "energy." Find the center of this area and press with a finger or thumb. The pressure should be no more than is comfortable for the patient and should last between five and ten seconds, occasionally longer, and can be repeated two or three times during the treatment in any one spot. This pressure point can correspond to a place in the body where life force energy is blocked, sluggish, or imbalanced and these blockages can sometimes move quite quickly when this pressure technique is applied. The patient may feel some sudden changes within: tingling sensations, becoming more relaxed, etc. The therapist may also feel things change and even the atmosphere in the room might feel different in a very short time. If anything unpleasant is experienced do not over-stimulate this point but carry on with the normal treatment and things will settle down quickly. You can come back to the same point later or in another treatment.

Fingertip pinch

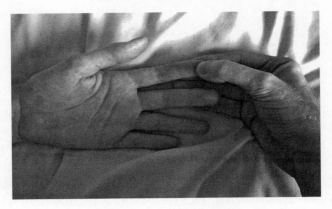

Figure 5   Finger pinch

This technique was mentioned earlier; it is a great way to stimulate the healing process. It can be included in a full treatment when you are treating the fingers and you can recommend that your clients use it themselves every day.

All the above techniques need to be practiced as much as possible on your own hands. You can do no harm with reflexology; it is a perfectly safe technique to use if you always follow correct instructions and use a light massage technique until you have some experience of the whole technique. It is a very enjoyable therapy to practice and receive and much fun can be had in learning and applying the techniques with friends and family. It is really great to learn in a class with others or with a friend or partner when you can practice on each other!

Reading the hands

When you inspect the hands during the first treatment you should be careful to notice certain things that are telltale signs of what areas you need to concentrate on during the treatment. When you look at the hands for the first time what is the very first impression you get? Do they look tired, fat, thin, pale, red, deformed? What condition is the skin in? Is it dry, sweaty, cracked? Is it the same all over? When you touch and massage the hands how do they react? Do they tense up or relax straight away? Do they feel stiff or without vitality and energy? When you massage certain areas do they feel, tense, puffy, inflamed, or lacking vitality? Can you feel anything under the skin like granules or grainy deposits? Do these break up under gentle massage or stubbornly remain? All these indications tell you about two things: the condition of the patient's body and the condition of the patient's mind. They also show you how well the client is as well as how unwell!

All these indications tell us that there is something going on inside the patient's body and/or mind that is reflected in the hands. As we know, different parts of the hands relate to different parts of the body so hard skin on the top of the thumb might be found on someone who is prone to headaches. Soft or tender skin on the upper part of the palm might be present in someone prone to chest infections or asthma. There are no rules as to what type of skin condition relates to what illness or physical weakness. We can only use them as a broad indication that some corresponding part of the body is in need.

During the treatment you can spend a little longer on those areas of the hands that seem to be lacking vitality, have hard or tender skin, etc. When you feel they are ready you can also encourage the patient to gently massage these areas for a few minutes twice a day between each treatment. However, you must stress "gently" and if there is a strong "detox" reaction then they should stop until this passes. You can also suggest they try to remove any hard skin: soaking their hands in warm water once a day and performing a few simple exercises afterwards. This might involve clockwise and anti-clockwise wrist rotations, clenching the fists tight for a few seconds then relaxing. They can gently massage their hands as well but again only gently. A very helpful and simple technique to help the healing process is to pinch the tip of each finger and thumb, hold the pressure for 10 seconds then release and tell the patient to do this two or three times per day, preferably when they are relaxed. Too much stimulation of the reflexes, especially in the first few weeks of treatment, can cause sickness, sweating, increased urination, and other side effects. In rare cases this can cause the client to cease treatment believing it to be a source of further illness instead of helping their condition! So again, start slowly and gently and encourage healing don't force it.

If you gradually learn to read the hands you will become very good at understanding your clients. All the indications that the hands report to you are valuable information that you need to assimilate and remember. If you are able to make notes on the state and condition of the hands during or before each treatment and compare the improvements that take place with the improvements that take place in the patient's body and mind you will be amazed at the obvious correlation. Some people are able to see into a person's mind and potential through palm reading, so this indicates that an open hand is like an open mind and the mind is the source of all illness and health. If we become good healers maybe we can develop a special kind of hand reflexology and learn to transmit healing energy to the patient on more subtle levels. We do not want to be fortune-tellers but we do need to use every opportunity to heal and help others.

You have to be careful not to alarm the patient with the signs and indications that the hands report. This can only depress and worry someone who might already be struggling to cope with a difficult illness. If in doubt, always be quiet. However, if you think that one of your patients should seek medical advice, tell them. Also, what you see in the hands might not indicate an immediate problem, just the early warning signs.

Self treatment

Some books go into detail about the various techniques of self-treatment. If you have a choice it is generally better to receive a reflexology treatment from someone else than to treat yourself. If there is no one you can turn to then by all means treat yourself. The main reason why self-treatment is inferior is the lack of comfort and the inability to relax during treatment. If you want to continue with self-treatment try 10 minutes reflexology on each hand every day for a week. Use the different techniques described in this book for treating others and adapt them yourself for self-treatment or learn the "10-minute technique" explained later in this book. As long as you give the whole of the hand a thorough going over, either using fingers, thumbs, knuckles, palms, or fists, then your self-treatment will be very effective. Also use the pinch and hold technique on the tip of each finger and thumb: this in itself can be very effective. Don't overdo it – after the first week cut the treatments down to every other day then every third day in the third week then once or twice a week thereafter. You may experience a big improvement to your state of physical and mental health. Keep the treatments up and this should continue.

As mentioned, there is no substitute for experience in becoming an accomplished reflexologist. At the beginning it may seem that there is too much to learn but if you learn a little and practice a little every day you will easily be able to complete your first full treatment within a few weeks, even earlier if you apply more effort. Obviously you will not be able to practice professionally without completing an appropriate course of study but you will be able to bring great benefit to friends and family who will be queuing up to take advantage of your new-found skills. There is a great sense of achievement and joy in seeing the results of a good treatment. This sense of accomplishment that you are doing something creative and meaningful with your time can be a real fuel encouraging you to improve and advance your skills further.

4

The hand reflexes

The following diagrams and text show in detail all the major reflexes on the hands. Gaining an accurate understanding of how the human anatomy is reflected in the reflexes is the key to good reflexology. The major reflexes like the head, spine, lungs, intestines, etc are quite easy to locate and memorize; however, it will seem at first as though there is a lot of information to digest. You do not need to memorize all that is shown before being able to practice successful reflexology. You can refer back to these guides as you continue learning the practical techniques. Then as you become more accomplished and confident you can deepen your knowledge by trying to memorize where the more intricate reflexes are located.

It is recommended then that the reader uses a comprehensive guide to anatomy and physiology to gain detailed knowledge where required. Such knowledge is essential if you wish to practice professionally and will form a key part of any practitioners' course. However, if you are happy to practice on friends and family the simple explanations that follow are more than adequate. Some bodily functions or organs are so well known that they need no explanation, whereas others are so complex that a full explanation would be impossible in a book of this nature. Also, many of the reflexes relating to different parts or bodily systems overlap. So an explanation of a particular system, like the nervous, lymphatic, or pulmonary system is given in the most appropriate place possible.

Reflexes – head and neck area

THE ENDOCRINE AND REPRODUCTIVE SYSTEMS

The main endocrine glands are the pituitary, thyroid, parathyroid, and adrenal glands, the ovary and testes, the placenta, and part of the pancreas. The endocrine system is made up of various glands, which secrete different types of hormones direct into the bloodstream. Through hormones they control the chemical composition, function, and stasis or balance of the body. Hormones are very potent chemical substances, and once they are produced they are carried around the body to different organs or tissues, which "recognize" or respond to them and subsequently alter their function or structure according to the type of hormone present. Every organ and tissue in the body is controlled by very complex chemical actions and reactions. Chemically the body is in a constant state of flux or inner motion and the endocrine system serves to control and balance all this inner activity.

Pituitary – sometimes referred to as the master endocrine gland. It is about the size of a pea and attached to the hypothalamus at the base of the skull. It secretes various important hormones.

Hypothalamus – Controls body temperature, hunger, water balance, and sexual function. It is also the center of cooperation or communication between the hormone and autonomic nervous system.

REMAINING HEAD REFLEXES

Ears and inner ear – The inner ear or "labyrinth" is a system of cavities and ducts that form the organs of hearing and balance, including the Eustachian tube, which connects the middle ear to the pharynx.

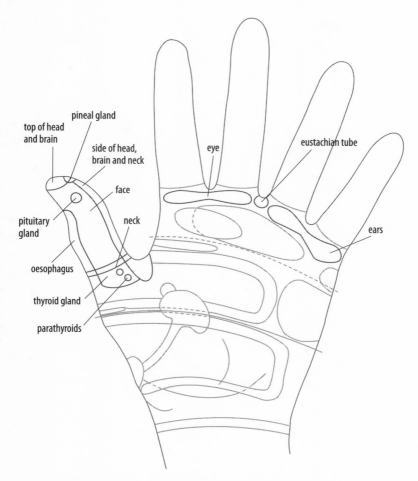

Figure 6 Reflexes for the head and neck

Reflexes – thoracic region

RESPIRATORY AND CIRCULATORY SYSTEMS

Our blood flows one way around the body over one thousand times a day. It provides all the major organs with what they need to function effectively, enables the immune system to operate,

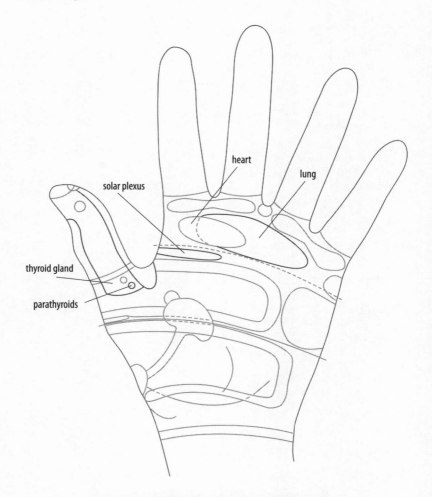

heart

solar plexus

lung

thyroid gland

parathyroids

Figure 7   Reflexes for the thoracic area

and continually removes and expels toxins. Blood is vitally oxygenated in the lungs and travels from the left side of the heart to all parts of the body, constantly regenerating and feeding the vital organs on the way back to the heart. The blood is "cleaned" and what toxins exist are removed along the way and the process begins again. Red blood cells carry oxygen around the body and white blood cells fight disease and infection, cleaning the blood and body of impurities. The production of white blood cells is increased during times of illness or infection. The respiratory and cardiac systems are very closely related, almost like two ends of a seesaw. When one is put under pressure by physical exertion the other responds and vice versa, until they find a balance that supplies the body with the amount of oxygen and rate of blood flow that it needs to continue.

Bronchial tree – A branching system of tubes from the base connection with the trachea to the tips of the bronchi and bronchioles, the smallest "branches," which open into the alveoli. There the gas exchange takes place with the blood capillaries surrounding them, oxygen going into the blood and waste gases being released for expulsion through exhalation.

Diaphragm – A thin dome-shaped muscle that separates the thoracic and abdominal cavities, playing a major role in respiration by stretching and expanding the lungs downwards upon inhalation.

OTHER REFLEXES IN THIS AREA

Thymus – Part of the immune system. Its main function is during infancy and before puberty. It controls the growth and development of a major part of the immune system.

Thyroid and parathyroid – Part of the endocrine system. The two main lobes of the thyroid gland mainly regulate the metabolic rate of the body, including mental and physical development. Excessive amounts or lack of thyroid hormones leads to ill-health. Behind or slightly within the thyroid are the parathyroid glands; these produce the hormones that control the distribution of calcium and phosphate in the body.

Solar plexus – Part of the nervous system. A complex and densely packed area of nerves forming part of the autonomic system located high in the back of the abdomen. A sensitive and important reflex for helping the whole body and mind relax.

Reflexes – abdominal area

DIGESTIVE SYSTEM

Our digestive system transforms our food and drink into simple nutritional forms that the various bodily functions require to sustain them. Ingestion is the first part of the process, which ends with the secretion of waste. In between there is a complex

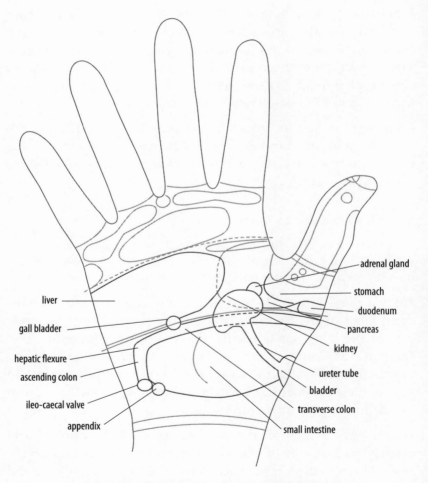

Figure 8   Reflexes for the abdominal area

process of breaking down the food and drink and absorbing what is required ready for use.

Esophagus/cardiac sphincter – The esophagus leads from the back of the mouth to the stomach and is lined with a mucus membrane that helps to lubricate the passage of food into the stomach. The cardiac sphincter is a ring of muscle, which controls entry into the stomach.

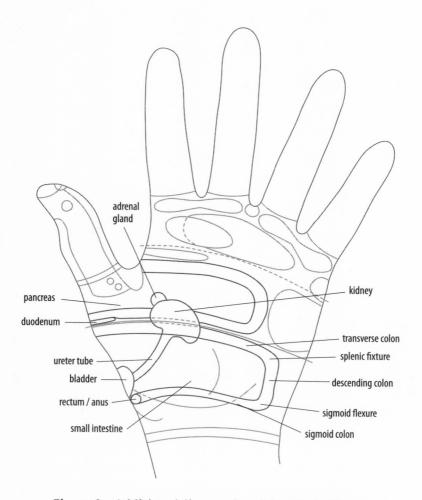

Figure 9   Additional diagram for abdominal reflexes

Stomach/pyloric sphincter – The stomach lies mainly to the left side of the body and forms a large muscular sack, which transforms food by chemically and mechanically blending and homogenizing it into a creamy substance known as chime. The pyloric sphincter is located at the exit to the stomach and is similar to the cardiac sphincter. Between them they control the amount of food entering and leaving the stomach.

Liver – Situated in the upper right side of the abdomen the liver produces bile for digestion, which drains into the gall bladder before being released into the duodenum. The liver also regulates blood sugar, removes excess amino acids, and stores and metabolizes fats, proteins, and carbohydrates. It also acts to detoxify the body and produces various other important chemicals.

Gall bladder – Under the right side of the liver, the gall bladder stores bile for use in digestion.

Pancreas – Found behind the stomach it forms and releases pancreatic juices into the duodenum through the pancreatic duct. Within the pancreas are groups of cells known as "Islets of Langerhans," which secret insulin and glucagon hormones into the bloodstream.

Small intestine – The first part of the small intestine is the duodenum, which stretches from the stomach to the jejunum – the second part of the system. It receives bile and pancreatic juices to help the process of digestion. The jejunum leads to the ileum, the lowest of the three parts of the small intestine, which ends in the ileo-cecal valve, which controls entry into the large intestine and prevents back flow into the ileum.

Appendix – A short tube with no obvious important purpose, attached to the digestive system close to the junction of the small and large intestine. There is some secretion into the large intestine, which helps to lubricate digestion and it also contains lymphatic material for the immune system.

Large intestine – About five feet in length it surrounds the small intestine by ascending, transversing, and descending on the left side of the body. The junctions between these three parts are called the hepatic flexure, splenic flexure, and sigmoid flexure respectively. The sigmoid flexure leads into the rectum and then the anus. All along the route that digested food takes, the necessary nutrients, vitamins, minerals, fats, etc are absorbed through the walls of the small and large intestine. Those nutrients, like fats, that require longer to digest are broken down and absorbed into the body in the large intestine. Those that can be assimilated more quickly are dealt with earlier on in the process, in the small intestine, the stomach and even in the esophagus.

OTHER REFLEXES IN THIS AREA

Adrenals – Part of the endocrine system. Covering the upper part of each kidney the adrenal glands produce adrenaline and corticosteroid hormones. Adrenaline affects the muscles, circulation, and sugar levels within the body and corticosteroid is a type of steroid.

MAIN PARTS OF THE URINARY SYSTEM

Kidneys – The kidneys cleanse the blood of soluble impurities and toxins, principally urea from the blood, and regulate water and mineral balance. The nephrons within the kidney filter the blood then reabsorb water and selected substances back into the blood.

Ureter – This tube connects the kidneys with the bladder and transmits the urine.

Bladder – Contains urine before urination.

Reflexes – pelvic area

Sciatic and pelvic area – The sciatic nerve is the main nerve of the leg. It is the largest nerve in the body and runs from the lower end of the spine down behind the thigh.

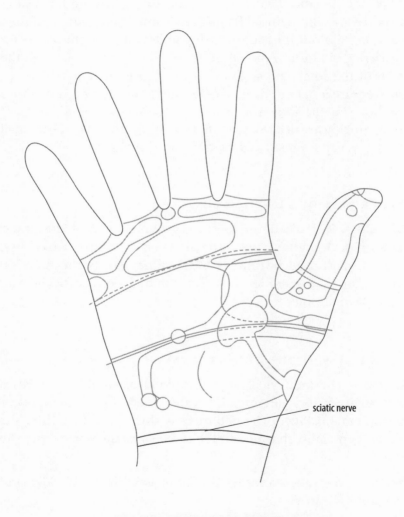

sciatic nerve

Figure 10 Reflexes for the pelvic area

Reflexes – reproductive organs

Ovaries – The female reproductive organs containing follicles that produce ova and steroid hormones in regular cycles.

Testes – The male reproductive glands producing spermatozoa and the male hormone testosterone.

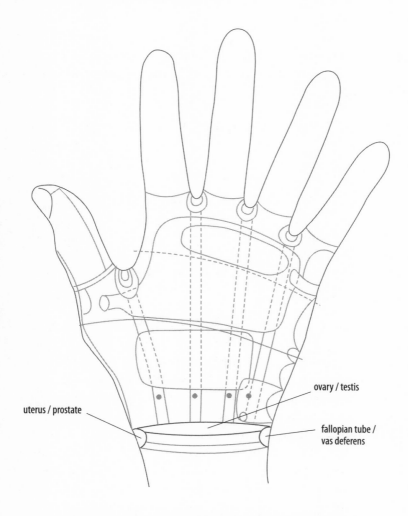

uterus / prostate

ovary / testis

fallopian tube / vas deferens

Figure 11   Reflexes for the reproductive organs

Uterus – Located in the central pelvic cavity in females it functions to nourish and protect the fetus during pregnancy.

Prostate – Found at the base of the bladder in males and opening into the urethra it produces fluid to carry and protect sperm.

Fallopian tubes – These connect the ovaries with the cavity of the uterus and transport the ova from the ovaries to the uterus during ovulation.

Urethra – The tube that expels urine from the bladder to the outside, ending at the tip of the penis in men and just within the vulva in women.

Vas deferens – These carry semen from the prostate to the urethra.

Reflexes – the spine

The spine consists of thirty-three vertebrae divided into five sections. It is the central support of the body and a main constituent in the nervous and skeletal system.

THE NERVOUS SYSTEM

The nervous system is a vast network of cells specifically designed to transmit nerve impulses or "information" to and from all areas of the body in order to bring about, monitor, and control all bodily activities, from the smallest adjustments at the microscopic level to the functions of all the major organs. It is the body's information highway.

The nervous system has three main parts, the central nervous system, the peripheral nervous system, and the autonomic nervous system. The central nervous system is responsible for the integration of all nervous activities, like a central mainframe computer. Its main components are the brain and spinal cord within the spinal column. The peripheral nervous system is all the other parts of the whole nervous system other than the central nervous system and this includes the cranial and spinal nerves. The autonomic nervous system is part of the peripheral system. It controls those parts of the body, over which the conscious mind has no regular or direct control, those parts of the body that need no conscious effort to work, for example the beating of the heart, sweating, intestinal movement, and the growth,

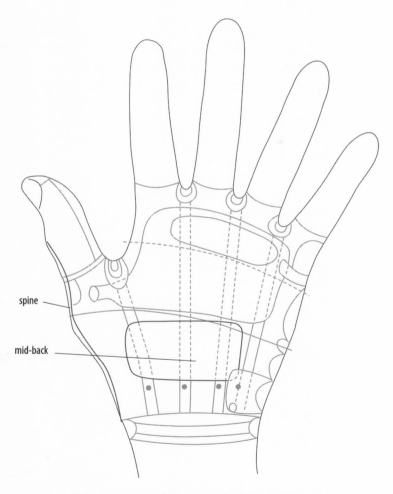

spine

mid-back

Figure 12   Reflexes for the spine

development, and ageing of the body. The autonomic system is again divided into two: the sympathetic nervous system and the parasympathetic system. It is through the autonomic nervous system that many people believe reflexology works.

Reflexes – the outer body

MUSCULAR AND SKELETAL SYSTEM

The skeletal system gives the body form and a rigid and strong framework allowing mobility and it also serves to protect and support vital organs. The main quality of muscle fiber is that it has the ability to contract producing movement or force.

Ribs, sternum, clavicle, and scapular – The sternum is better known as the chest bone and the clavicle and scapular as the collar bone and shoulder blade respectively.

Hands – Running form the wrist to the fingers the main bones are the carpals, metacarpals, and phalanges.

Feet – Running from the ankle to the toes the main bones are the tarsals, metatarsals, and phalanges.

Arms – Upper arm bone or humerus. Lower arm bones or radius (largest) and ulna.

Legs – Thigh bone or femur. Lower leg bones or tibula (largest) and fibula.

Reflexes – the lymphatic system

LYMPHATIC SYSTEM

Forming a major part of the body's immunity, the lymphatic system is made up of a network of lymph nodes and channels. Lymph, which is made up of proteins, electrolytes, and water,

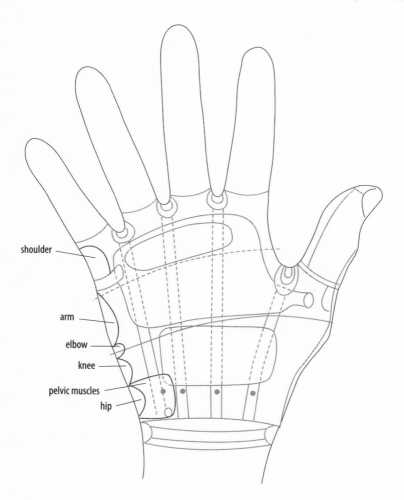

shoulder

arm

elbow

knee

pelvic muscles

hip

Figure 13   Reflexes for the outer body

is carried from tissue fluids to the bloodstream. The lymphatic vessels or channels lead to two large channels, the right lymphatic duct and the thoracic duct, which return the lymph to the bloodstream. This system needs the movement of the body, as well as respiration and gravity, to work most effectively; it works to fight disease and infection and remove everyday toxins from the body.

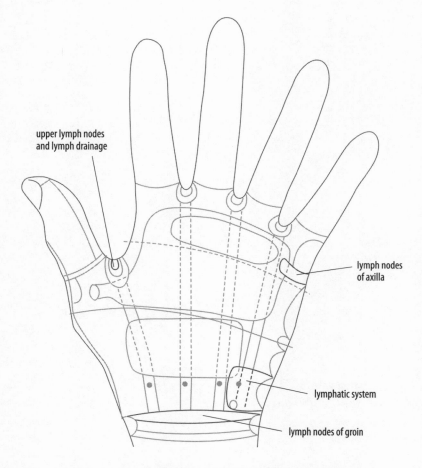

upper lymph nodes
and lymph drainage

lymph nodes
of axilla

lymphatic system

lymph nodes of groin

Figure 14   Reflexes for the lymphatic system

Upper lymphatics – Mainly located in the head, neck, armpits, and central chest area.

Lower lymphatics – Mainly located around the solar plexus/stomach area, spleen, groin, and behind the knees.

5

A full treatment

nitially it is helpful to pace yourself well and not take on too much, perhaps just a few treatments per week is a good start. Eventually you may be able to do several per day depending on your own strength, although quality is always better than quantity. If you are treating someone else they need to be able to relax properly during the treatment so they can either be lying down or sitting in a comfortable chair, preferably with some kind of head rest so they can lean back and completely relax into the treatment. To work the various reflexes you can sit in front of them with their hand resting on a cushion in your lap or on a small table. Their hand and arm should be completely relaxed. Once you have finished treating one hand you will need to move around to the other side of the patient to treat the other. You may also want to move your position while you are treating one hand: you might start by facing the patient and then move around to sit by the side of the patient. You need to find your own way: one that is most comfortable for you and the client and feels most effective in terms of covering the reflex areas. Treating the hands is not done with great effort and the different types of movement do not require great strength. The best reflexologists are not the strongest, so don't think that bulging muscles and strenuous massage are required.

You can practice the main hand movements on your own hands or feet as mentioned previously. This helps you to feel what they are like and to determine how much pressure is required. Of course when you are treating others you do not want to hurt them so you need to be prepared to adapt to the needs of the individual. Some hands are very sensitive and if the patient is ill and has never had reflexology before the first few treatments may need to be very light. Some parts of the hand may be much more sensitive than others, so again the first treatment should be simply exploratory and you should note those areas that need a light touch. This also helps you to recognize progress in the treatment, as when the sensitive areas become less painful this is a good sign that the corresponding physical anatomy is reacting well to the treatment.

Firm or gentle touch

Reflexologists generally use a combination of light touch and deep massage. Some reflexologists never use a deep massage technique because they feel it is ineffective and can, if used without thought, cause pain and discomfort to the patient. In some Chinese forms of reflexology deep massage is the only technique used along with even more brutal techniques using short sticks to press deep into the sole of the foot. There is no doubt that such treatments are painful and the cries and shouts of patients can often be heard outside the clinic! However, there is also no doubt that such treatments are very effective and have been for thousands of years.

Modern western reflexology is not like this. Although deep massage can be applied using techniques like the knuckle press you should only use them when you are experienced. You should never use them if the patient experiences pain, although some discomfort is acceptable if the patient is genuinely accepting of this. When you get some experience of when to apply more pressure these deep massage techniques can be very effective if used sparingly. You would never use deep massage in the first or second treatment with a new client unless you are sure it is wise to do so. Some reflexologists only ever use a very light touch and this is also a very effective technique. It certainly allows the patient to relax well and seems to induce a really subtle and deep state of healing, particularly helpful for mental and emotional problems. As individual therapists you need to practice and find your own way of doing things. The way that naturally feels right to you is usually the best and most effective. And there is no reason for you not to use a different technique with different types of patient according to their needs and your experience and confidence.

There are several schools of thought on the order in which the various reflexes should be treated. The following is one of the most well known and widely used. But that does not mean it is necessarily any more effective than others. Once you have mastered the basics you can look at other schools of thought and decide for yourselves through experience and the results of your practice what to use and what to discard.

It is easier to learn the reflexes for each bodily system while also learning about the system itself. So it is worth referring regularly to the explanations in Chapter 4. You will also need to remind yourselves of where the more intricate reflexes are located. As some of the reflexes for different physiological systems overlap, rather than doubling up on some, you can make changes to the sequence of treatment to make it slightly quicker and more efficient but just as effective. But it is important to learn the basics well before you do this. As a general rule, if you cover all of the reflexes in one treatment then this is the main requirement. In the beginning if you get the order wrong or forget to complete the sequence of reflexes for a system you can just add them on at the end of the treatment or at an appropriate point mid-session, and this will generally not adversely affect the quality of results.

The following movements for stretching and relaxing the hands are always used at the beginning of a full treatment to help the client relax physically and mentally and help the therapist prepare mentally and physically. Some reflexologists also use these hand techniques during and after a treatment. The sequence you choose to relax the hands is not too important.

The way the various movements are presented in the following text is an effective sequence but your experience may show you otherwise. If you think of some new movements try them on yourself or a friend to see of they are comfortable and useful. It is important to gain some experience of giving and receiving these warm-up movements. Always begin gently then there is no fear of injury and as always be especially careful with sensitive or "new" hands.

Some of the warm-up movements can be used throughout the rest of the treatment and can form part of the treatment. In fact, if you only have a short amount of time, say 10 to 15 minutes, they can be used to give a short treatment. For example, this could be practiced on someone who has just come home from work to help them wind down or first thing in the morning to help them wake up! This is an excellent method for relaxing and de-stressing anyone in only a short time. Work on one hand at a time and keep the other warmly wrapped in a small towel.

Reflexologists tend to develop their own style of warm-up procedure so try the above exercises on a few friends to see what they like and to see what you feel is most helpful. But don't get stuck in a rut with one set procedure. With experience you will get to know which clients or patients like which kind of warm-up and how much pressure to apply during the treatment. Also, don't be too light with your touch techniques – sometimes an almost vigorous warm-up and a firm touch during the treatment might really suit a particular patient. Experience and confidence will be your guides.

Warm-up techniques

Gently hold the hand and forearm as shown above, rotate the wrist a few times one way then the other, and then gently push the hand away from you to stretch the muscles and do the same in the opposite direction. The main consideration is not to stretch too much or rotate too fast; do everything slowly and gently especially on the first treatment.

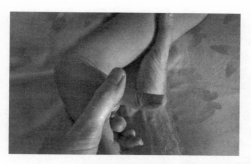

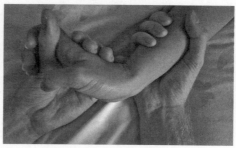

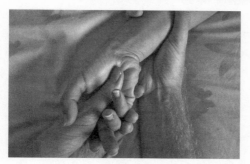

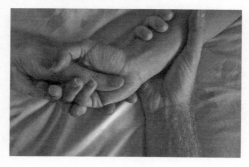

Figures 15a-15d   Warm-up exercises 1 and 2

Gently but firmly hold the hand and forearm as shown above and pull, then relax and pull again, do this a few times.

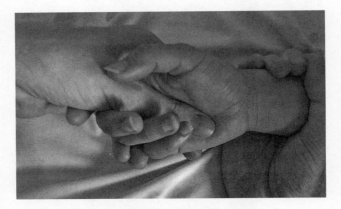

Figure 16　Warm-up exercise 3

Cup the patient's hand in yours, gently squeeze, then relax and repeat a few times. During the squeeze you can gently move your hands in opposite directions – up and down and forward and backward.

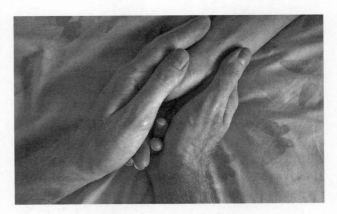

Figure 17　Warm-up exercise 4

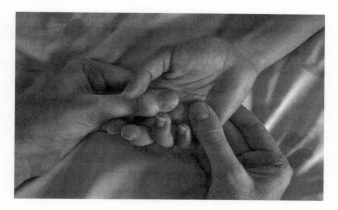

Figure 18   Warm-up exercise 5

Use your thumbs and forefingers to gently hold the hands and find the bones; work across the palm from one side to another, gently moving the bones up and down and from side to side.

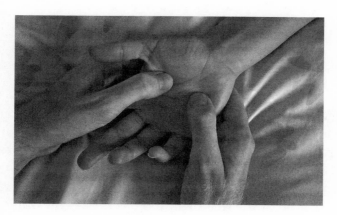

Figure 19   Warm-up exercise 6

Use your thumbs one after another to gently press the reflexes all over the hands and fingers (front and back), using a light, quick, and gentle touch or press.

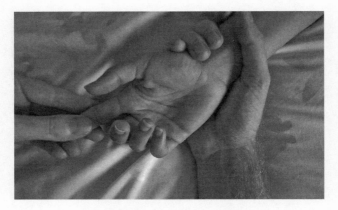

Figure 20   Warm-up exercise 7

Finally, gently but firmly pull each finger and thumb while allowing your grip to slide toward the top of each finger and thumb. When you reach the tip gently pinch and hold for a few seconds. You can repeat this at the end of the treatment holding each pinch for about 10 seconds.

The main part of the treatment

This section shows how to complete a full treatment. As you begin each section refer back to the diagrams showing the location of each reflex with its associated bodily part or function. There are some specific techniques for treating particular reflexes explained below. Generally, as long as you cover all the reflexes in one section of the treatment there is no specific order that is more effective than another. In your first few treatments you are bound to forget to treat some reflexes and this is fine, no harm can be done. If you learn each section of reflexes methodically within a few weeks you will be able to give a full treatment without referring to the book. This is a great feeling and shows that you are really deepening your knowledge, understanding, and experience of reflexology. In fact, the sooner you can give treatments without referring to the book the better. Then you can begin to really tune in to the patient and develop your own style of reflexology. It is not a race but the quicker you learn the basics the quicker you can relax and start to listen to what the patient needs and also develop your own intuitive healing abilities. If you have or develop a genuine wish to help others without a strong sense of self-importance or pride as a healer then you will definitely become an accomplished reflexologist and a real source of help for others.

The fingers and thumbs – the head and neck

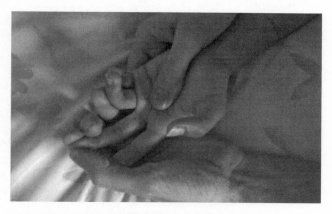

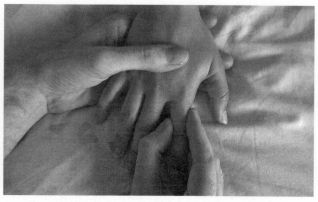

Figure 21   Head and neck reflexes 1

You will know by now that the thumb and finger reflexes correlate to the head and neck area of the body. Beginning at the very tip of each finger you treat the sinus reflexes. You do this by simply using the nibbling or "walking" thumb massage. You need to support each finger with your own fingers so that it does not bend under the gentle pressure of the massage. As with most of the various treatment sections, where the same reflexes exist on both hands you begin with one hand and then treat the same reflex on the other. However, some reflexologists prefer to treat one hand almost completely while keeping the other warmly but loosely wrapped up in a small towel. With experience you can decide which is more effective.

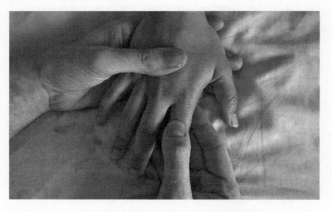

Figure 22   Head and neck reflexes 2

We use the same technique to work the front and back of each finger and thumb. The side of each finger can be treated in the same way or using the index finger to massage gently from the top to the bottom. The reflexes on the inside of the fingers are often quite sensitive, so a gentle touch is especially important and you must not bend the finger by applying too much pressure.

Do not skimp on massaging the fingers, as they are at least as important as the rest of the hands. A healing response is stimulated in each of the 10 zones of the body by massaging the fingers.

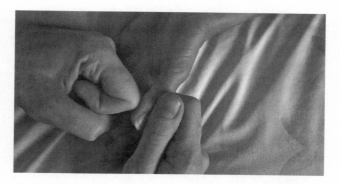

Figure 23   Head and neck reflexes 3

By using these techniques thoroughly you will have covered nearly all the main reflexes for the head and neck. By referring back to the relevant reflex chart you will see that there are so many important areas treated, especially those relating to the brain, that you may find the patient is already very relaxed and some healing energy is really starting to flow.

One of these very important reflexes is the pituitary gland and it is found within the brain reflex on the thumb. Using the knuckle of the index finger press in, rotate and lift. If you have located it correctly the patient may feel a little sharp pain. Do not cause too much pain by over-stimulating it. Do this on both thumbs.

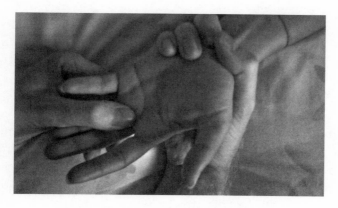

Figure 24   Head and Neck Reflexes 4

Moving on to the area just below the base of each finger, use the thumb to massage these reflexes relating to the eyes and ears. You can use the fingers of the same hand to support the back of the patient's hand. You will be working in a horizontal line across the top of the palm.

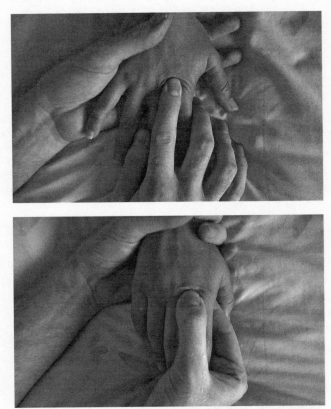

Figure 25   Upper lymphatic reflexes

The final area in this section is the upper lymphatic reflexes on the top of the hand. They are stimulated using the finger or thumb massage technique. Work the appropriate area shown on the diagram in lines from the fingers toward the wrist, especially concentrating on the soft area between the bones. You will feel the bones move apart slightly as you apply pressure and these areas might be sensitive, so be careful not to apply too much pressure on the first or second treatment.

This is also a good point to treat the whole of the top of the hand if you wish by simply using the same technique to carry on the massage up to the lymphatic reflexes on the wrists. Do not go down the side of the hand as these areas are covered later. This whole area helps the lymphatic system and from zone therapy we know that many other bodily functions and systems will be stimulated and relaxed.

Upper palm – thoracic area

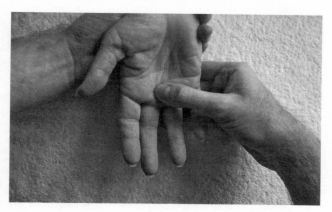

Figure 26   Thoracic reflexes 1

From the reflex charts you will see that some major organs and glands are located in this area and many medical conditions relating to the heart, lungs, and thyroid, for example, respond well to treating these reflexes. As shown in the figure we use the thumb massage technique. This area is often toughened from manual work so we might have to apply a little more pressure than normal.

We can work in vertical lines from bottom to top or from left to right using our right and then left thumb. Alternatively we can work in diagonal lines one way and then the other. As long as we cover the whole area that is the main thing.

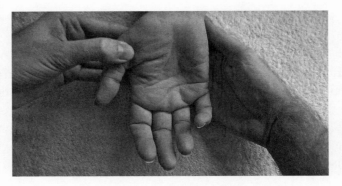

Figure 27   Thoracic reflexes 2

For the thyroid, parathyroid, and base of the neck reflexes treat the area around the base of the thumbs and repeat this two or three times. This may be a sensitive area so proceed with caution with a new patient.

Mid palm – abdominal area

If you look at the detailed reflex charts you will see that most of the reflexes for the digestive system are contained within this area. This area is also the most complicated in terms of the number of reflexes and the way they often overlap. Some reflexology books present various complicated methods for methodically treating each reflex in a specific order.

This can be very effective but there is no research or anecdotal evidence to suggest it is any more effective than using a simple horizontal, vertical, and/or diagonal thumb walking technique to cover the whole area from top to bottom. Alternatively we can introduce some simple compromise that takes the best from the complicated and simple systems, as follows.

Starting with the liver reflex this takes up a substantial area on the patient's right hand as it is located on the right side of the body. The top of the liver is found just below the right lung reflex, we work from top to bottom and left to right in horizontal or diagonal lines. As we work down the liver reflex we will also begin to work the stomach, pancreas, and duodenum reflexes as they overlap in this area.

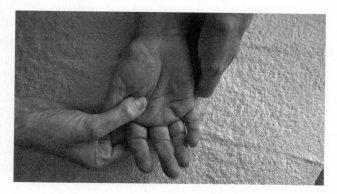

Figure 28   Abdominal reflexes 1

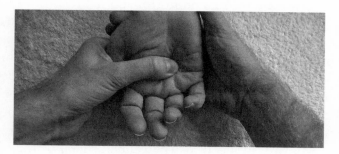

Figure 29   Abdominal reflexes 2

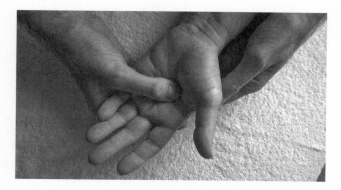

Figure 30   Abdominal reflexes 3

Once we have worked the liver we need to go back and locate the gall bladder reflex. It is usually located at the bottom of the liver reflex directly in line with the patient's third finger. You can press and massage it in a circular motion or just press gently and hold for 5-10 seconds. Some reflexologists do not treat the gall bladder separately at all but feel that simply working the liver is enough, which it often is.

The next important reflexes in this area are the stomach, pancreas, duodenum, and spleen. The reflex chart shows the area we need to cover to treat them effectively. Beginning with the patient's right hand we work that area to the right of the liver reflexes. It is important to avoid the liver area as over-stimulating the reflexes is never beneficial. Then, moving to the patient's left hand we treat the reflex area for the stomach, pancreas, and duodenum toward the mid point from both directions. The right half covers part of the stomach, the spleen, and part of the colon. Treating this area we will also cover the main part of the kidneys and adrenal glands, although we will cover these reflexes in more detail further on.

The lower part of this area includes the reflexes for the small intestine, ileo-cecal valve, appendix, and large intestine. All the hands you treat will be a slightly different size and shape so the reflexes will vary in location. The general shape of the hand is the clue to locating them and the diagrams given throughout this book are an accurate guide on which to base your treatments.

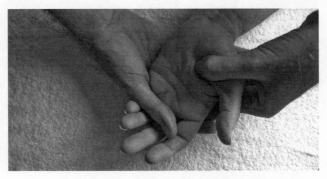

Figure 31   Abdominal reflexes 4

The best way to treat this area of the hands is in the general direction in which the intestines work. So we begin working the small intestine going from right to left in horizontal lines. We can work right across this area from top to bottom before moving on to the small intestine reflexes in the other hand. Once this is complete we return to the patient's right hand to begin working the large intestine from the bottom left hand corner of this area. At this point we will find the ileo-cecal valve reflex, which we can press and hold for a few seconds before beginning to work up and across on the large intestine reflex. Moving to the patient's left hand we continue until we reach the side of the hand and then work down the remaining area of the reflex down to the sigmoid flexure and anus. The last reflexes to be covered in this area are for the urinary system and include the kidneys, adrenals, ureter, and bladder. Most of these reflexes will have already been stimulated if you have followed the previous instructions. However, most reflexologists like to cover them again and more accurately with this method. If you are worried about over-stimulation then when you cover these areas in previous sections use a lighter touch and again, when treating them specifically, do the same.

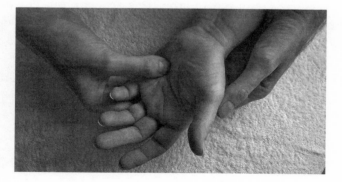

Figure 32   Abdominal reflexes 5

Next treat the kidneys; the adrenals are located directly on and above the kidneys and both can be treated at the same time. Work the patient's right and then left kidney, then the right and then left ureter, and finally the right and left bladder. The bladder reflex curves around the inside of the hand as shown in the photograph above and can appear like an area of "slack" or puffy skin. It can also be sensitive, so a light touch is used initially.

Base of hand – pelvic area

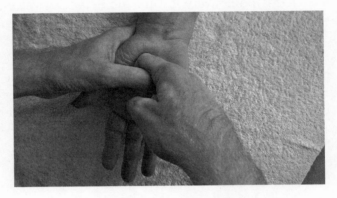

Figure 33   Pelvic Reflexes

Often the most muscular area of the hand to work, so a little more pressure is required and the knuckle technique can be used if there is thick or hard skin or if you feel it is OK to work deeply. Simply press the knuckle in and slowly drag it across the reflex area in straight lines until all the area is covered.

This area may be especially sensitive in people with a physical problem in the corresponding pelvic region. You can work from side to side or top to bottom to cover this area.

Wrists – reproductive organs

The reflexes for all the reproductive organs are located around the wrist area (see reflex charts). These can often be quite sensitive so a gentle touch is required to begin with. Look at the reflex chart to see which areas need to be treated.

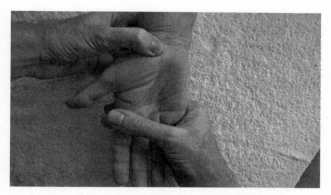

Figure 34   Reproductive organ reflexes

Inner edge – the spine

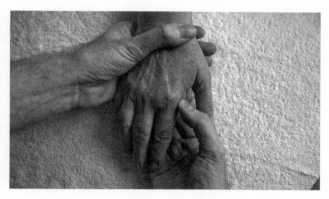

Figure 35   Spine reflexes

The spine reflex runs up the inner aspect of the hand and about half way up the thumb. Since it is such an important part of the nervous system, treating this reflex will have a beneficial effect on the whole body. We begin at the base of the reflex and work our way up following the line of the reflex shown in the diagram. The reflex is split, the left side of the spine being on the inside of the patient's left hand and the right side on the right hand. We can work each reflex several times, also working slightly to the left and then right of the main reflex to ensure we have covered it completely.

Outer edge – the outer body

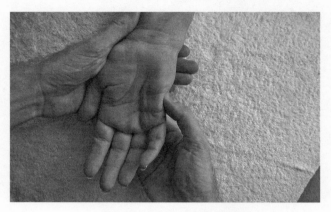

Figure 36   Outer body reflexes

The reflex diagram shows the outer aspect of the patient's hand, revealing the reflexes for the knee, hip, elbow, and shoulder, the hip reflex being the largest in this sequence and the shoulder reflex being just below the little finger.

Top of the hands – chest and circulation

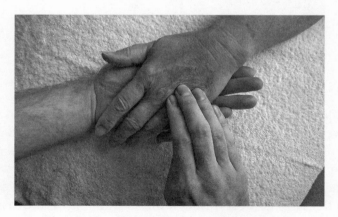

Figure 37   Chest and circulation reflexes

At this point we are beginning to bring the treatment to an end, having covered most of the reflexes that require treatment.

Toward the beginning of the treatment we covered this last area when treating the upper lymphatics, so only a light touch is now required to prevent over-stimulation, although you can work some reflexes a little more vigorously if there is a specific problem in the corresponding area of the body. You can work the top of the hand in a gentle way using three or four fingers of each hand to cover the whole area from the base of the patient's fingers to the wrists (see figure above).

Warm-down techniques

The last technique is really the first of the warm-down techniques. The others in this sequence can include some of the gentler warm-up techniques mentioned earlier and a general light massage over the whole of the hands. You will develop your own techniques in time, ones that are simply relaxing are the best. As well as being the perfect conclusion to the treatment they give the client a subtle hint that the treatment is nearly over.

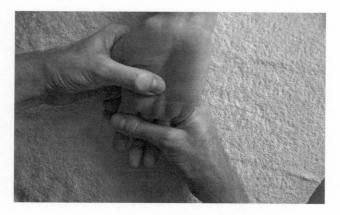

Figure 38   Warm-down techniques

Often the best way to end a treatment is to use the solar plexus breathing technique. Bend the fingers of one hand back slightly and press the solar plexus reflex; at the same time ask the patient to breathe in, hold this for a few seconds, then ask the patient to breathe out and release your press; repeat this two or three times on each hand. This is relaxing but also helps to wake the client up if they are asleep or drowsy.

This completes the treatment. If the patient is still asleep simply squeeze the hands gently or touch them on the shoulder but do allow them plenty of time to come around before sitting or standing up. There is no rush and the last thing you want to do is hurry one patient out and the next one in!

6

The 10-minute technique and zone therapy

The 10-minute technique

This chapter will teach you a simple 10-minute reflexology technique that you can practice every day on yourself or others to improve physical or mental health. You can also teach this technique to others if you think they would benefit from it. The key to success with this technique is to practice it every day. It's easy to find 10 minutes every day but it may be difficult to find 45 minutes for yourself to apply a full treatment. This 10-minute technique can even be more powerful than a full treatment once a week because we are stimulating the healing reflexes more regularly. Ideally though, the best method is a combination of both, for example, a full treatment once a week and the 10-minute technique once a day, or every other day if you do not have the time or it might be putting to much pressure on your body. This might especially be the case if you are ill. It is possible to overdo it with reflexology, so be gentle with yourself. Don't push too hard; start off gently and see how you feel. If you start experiencing overpowering detox symptoms, like going to the toilet very often, sweating, and feeling as if you have flu then ease up, make your treatments shorter or less frequent, or apply less pressure during the massage.

Another important point is don't do the 10-minute massage as well as the zone therapy techniques mentioned in the next chapter – that would be too intense. Try both out for a few days or weeks and see which works best for you; both are excellent methods for developing better health.

The sequence for the 10-minute treatment is similar to that for a full treatment, the main difference is that we work with less precision and more speed. Initially you might think that this makes for an inferior treatment and that assumption would be correct if you were only treating yourself for 10 minutes each week, but because we are repeating this technique each day the cumulative effect over a few days or weeks can be quite powerful. So don't be put off if you don't feel as good after 10 minutes as you would after forty-five! Wait for a few days at least before you judge the effectiveness of this type of treatment. This is a different approach to healing – a little more proactive than reactive, and it fits ideally in to the modern lifestyle and can work especially well for those personality types who are at their happiest in the business of daily life. We all have different capacities, skills, and tendencies: some people like to take life slowly and steadily and some people like to go full steam ahead. We all need to do a little of both sometimes to lead a well-balanced life but we need to know ourselves and work out what kind of relaxation or healing techniques are right for us. If you are a therapist you need to learn how to spot these personality traits in others and advise them accordingly. Often, when people are ill or overworked we tell them to rest and take time out, and this is generally good advice. Occasionally, however, it might be more beneficial to advise someone to be more active, and seek out new challenges and relationships. In these situations, and for the more dynamic personality type, the 10-minute technique can work really well! As mentioned, though, it can just be a great support to regular, full-length reflexology treatments.

Preparation for the 10-minute treatment is minimal: you can do it anywhere at any time, although if you choose the same time and place every day that can help you to get into a good habit and avoid missing a day. A natural pause in the day is good to find, like just before lunch, when you get home, just before bed, or get up 10 minutes earlier. You can do it on the bus or train, even while walking if your hands are free. All of these are possibilities. You need to try it out for yourself and see how you can fit it into your day. Some people find that the hand massage wakes them up and some people find it ideal before they go to bed, so find what works best for you. If you can find at least a few minutes before the massage to relax, that can really help, as reflexology works much better on a relaxed body and mind. You can also use this technique to help you cope with a stressful situation. If you know that you will be facing a difficult situation try to find 10 minutes about thirty minutes before the event and that will help you to feel relaxed and strong. Also, if something stressful happens out of the blue try to find a quiet place, sit down for a few minutes, and begin the 10-minute treatment; this will help you recover much faster, especially if you combine this with taking a homeopathic remedy or flower essence like Rescue Remedy. Drinking a few pints of filtered or mineral water each day, especially during the first week of self-treatment, can help the detox process and you can also combine this technique with a juice detox program. You can develop your own warm-up technique based on the procedures used during a full treatment: choose whichever you like best given the time you have available. A simple way to begin is to clench and hold your hands as a fist for a few seconds then relax, repeat this a few times, then keep all the muscles relaxed and shake your hands as if you were shaking water from them after washing. Also, you can rotate the wrists one way and then the other, then do the same with the thumbs, then use the fingers of one hand to rotate each finger of the other hand so that the joint at the knuckle is loosened. Any combination of the techniques and those mentioned earlier is fine. The main criterion is time: if you have it do a good warm-up, if you don't move into the main technique more quickly. Some people also find it helpful to soak their hands in warm water for a minute or two to relax all the muscles. If you have an aromatherapy oil to hand this can really add to the effectiveness of the treatment; use the right type of oil according to what effect you are trying to achieve (see Appendix 3 for a list of oils and their uses).

The actual techniques

1. Begin by pinching and holding the top of each finger and thumb, use as much pressure as you like without it becoming painful. If you are using the 10-minute technique at the start of the day you can be more dynamic and use more pressure and if you are using the technique to wind down at the end of the day you can use a more gentle approach. Pinch and hold the sides of the top of each finger and thumb for a few seconds and then the top and bottom as shown in the figures below.

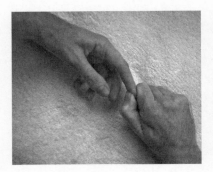 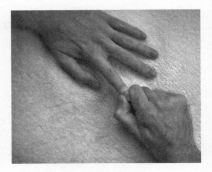

2. Then take each finger and thumb in turn and rub the sides and top vigorously between the thumb and first finger of the other hand; again use as much pressure as you can without hurting

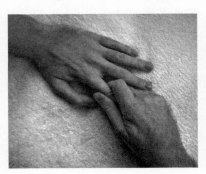 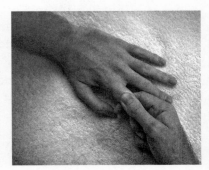

yourself. If you use too much pressure at this stage the muscles of the massaging hand will become too tired to continue to the end of the treatment! As your muscles become stronger you will be able to apply more pressure for longer. Don't spend too long, maybe 10 seconds on each finger or thumb.

3. Hold each finger firmly in turn at the base, again using the thumb and first finger, and pull up to the tip of the finger or thumb at the end and give a little pinch. Do this twice on each finger so that the top and bottom and sides are treated.

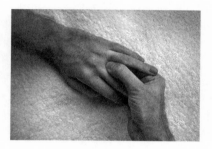

4. Next pinch and hold the area between the base of each finger and thumb and after a few seconds slowly pull away until you lose contact, then move on to the next. If you have time you can also massage this area a little. When you apply pressure, if the area is tender just hold it for a few seconds and the discomfort should lessen; if it doesn't then apply less pressure.

5. Moving to the back of the hands, use the fingers of one hand to support the other and the thumb of the supporting hand to massage the back of the supported hand from the wrist to the base of the fingers. You can be quite vigorous and apply plenty of pressure while moving the thumb in a circular motion all over the back of the hand. You can use the tip of the thumb to apply deep massage to the areas between the bones. If you have more time you can use the thumb walking technique to work from one side of the hand to the other or from the wrist to the base of the fingers.

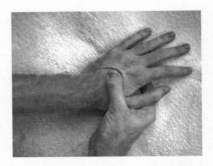

6. Then moving to the palms it can be helpful to roughly split the palm into three areas: the base of the palm and inner wrist, the top of the palm below the base of the fingers (corresponds to the ball of the foot), and the central area. The easiest method is to support one hand with the fingers of the other and use the thumb of the supporting hand to deeply massage firstly the upper palm, then the central area, and finally the base and inner wrist. Another method is to rest one hand on your thigh and apply pressure to the palm area using the knuckle of the first finger of the other hand. Apply as much pressure as you can comfortably bear and rotate the knuckle as you apply pressure; repeat this many times to cover the whole area of the palm. The knuckle technique seems to work best on the fleshy areas, where it is OK to apply more pressure. Don't use the knuckle technique on the inner wrist; a gentle thumb massage is all that is needed here.

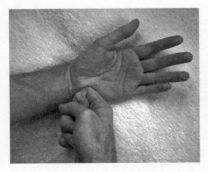
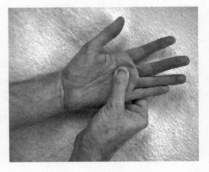

7. Finish the treatment with a simple pressure hold for 10 seconds, with your thumb in the center of each palm. Then repeat some of the warm-up exercises to finish, like clenching, holding, and releasing your fists and shaking the hands or just gently stroking each hand with the fingertips of the other hand.

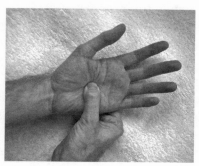

You can combine the 10-minute technique with some of the zone therapy techniques mentioned later. But don't overdo it; the healing process takes time and should not be rushed. It is much better to be gentle with yourself for the first few days and weeks and build up steadily. Too much reflexology can put a lot of pressure on your body, especially if you are ill. Everyone is different, though, so start off gently and if you feel ready to use a deeper massage or spend a little longer that's fine.

Although these techniques are ideal for people with busy lives the healing process cannot be rushed and if a busy life is creating or contributing to your health problems applying these techniques alone is not enough. You need to lead a balanced life: time for recreation, developing good relationships, helping others, etc, are as important as, if not more important than, a successful career or a high income. A good quality of life can create and support good mental and physical health. Good quality of life principally comes from a good quality of mind: if you have a positive and relaxed approach to life this is a great basis to begin a program of self-healing. Developing this approach to life can lead to certain decisions like a change of career or maybe accepting a drop in income to be able to spend more time with your family or on a project that is close to your heart. Sometimes, to help the healing process we just need to identify what it is that would make our life really worthwhile or meaningful; ask your heart! No one ever said on their deathbed, "Oh I wish I had spent more time in the office." Not everyone is in a position to change their career or accept a drop in income, and for many people with major responsibilities or challenging living conditions time to think or make choices for themselves is an impossible luxury. Whatever your situation you can make a decision to live positively; we all have a mind and we can take control and develop our inner qualities whatever our external situation. This takes determination, training, skill, and wisdom but the rewards can be limitless. One way to begin is to read some good books about training the mind (see Appendix 2). So a balanced life means using your time well, if possible finding time to relax, spending quality time with others, good diet, enjoyable exercise, and perhaps most importantly developing your mind. If you reach the end of your life wiser, more content, more kind, more at peace with yourself and more accepting of others, that must be a life well spent. You can use this yardstick each year: by the end of this year if you are a more whole and healthy human being then that must be a year well spent, if you are only materially richer then in reality this has little meaning. Human beings have such a special opportunity to develop themselves. Your evolution is in your own hands.

Zone therapy techniques

In this chapter we will learn some well-known zone therapy techniques that can be used alongside or instead of the reflexology techniques. As mentioned earlier, zone therapy developed in the West before reflexology and it is still a separate therapy today, although not as widespread as reflexology. The technique works on the principles that the body can be divided into 10 zones and applying pressure to one part of the body in a particular zone will have a beneficial effect on the other body parts within that zone. Zone therapists believe this works for two reasons. Firstly, science tells us that the body is an electromagnetic field and there are 10 main electric currents running through the body in line with the toes and fingers. Secondly, all the main meridians, the subtle life energy channels, either begin or end in either the feet or the hands. We cannot say for certain why zone therapy, reflexology, or acupressure work but we know from experience that they can contribute greatly to increased mental and physical health and vitality. This is a practical chapter with the aim of sharing those zone therapy techniques that can be easily learnt and are most effective. You can use one or two of the techniques as a help or boost to the 10-minute technique or regular reflexology sessions. You would not use all the various options together as that would be too much.

The first simple method is to pinch and hold the tip of each finger and thumb. The easiest way to apply strong pressure is to hold the tip of the finger between the thumb and knuckle of the first finger of the other hand. Apply as much pressure as you can reasonably bear without experiencing pain; a little discomfort is fine! Hold this for about 20 seconds on each finger. If you have more time, begin at the base of each finger and thumb, squeeze and hold for a few seconds, then release and move up slightly and repeat this many times until you reach the top of the finger or thumb, where you can hold for maybe 10 seconds or more. See the picture of the finger squeeze at the beginning of the 10-minute technique. Another way to do this technique is to use some strong elastic bands and wrap one around the top of each finger and thumb. Wrap them as tight as you can bear and leave them on for a few minutes at most and then transfer them to the other hand. This must be the easiest way to better health! You can even do it while you are watching TV. Repeat this technique two or three times a day. Obviously you must lessen the tension of the elastic bands if you feel it is harming the finger and if you are using the 10-minute technique perhaps only use the elastic bands once per day. As an alternative, some people like to use clothes pegs or perhaps you can think of another method of automatic zone therapy!

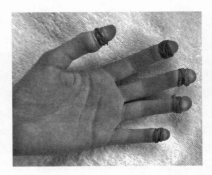

There are other methods to apply pressure to zones ending in the fingers. One way is to place one hand flat on the surface of a table and apply pressure to the top of each finger and thumb with the base of the other hand. You can apply a lot of pressure like this, so don't push too hard. Another method is again to lay one hand on a table, palm up, and apply pressure to the tip of each finger and thumb with the blunt end of a pencil, preferably one with a rubber tip. Apply as much pressure as feels OK, i.e. without experiencing pain, and hold this for maybe 15 seconds; if it feels OK to hold the pressure for longer that's fine, but no more than one minute per finger. With this method you can start at the base of the finger and work up, applying pressure for a few seconds each time.

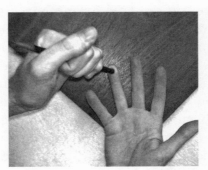

You can use zone therapy at any time, like the 10-minute hand reflexology technique it can be especially helpful when you are feeling tired or a bit low, before or after any stressful situation, if you have a few spare minutes at work before an important meeting, or your children are being very demanding. There are so many challenges in daily life that can be made easier with a few minutes of hand massage or zone therapy.

Another zone therapy method is to use a comb or brush on the palm or the back of each hand. Because all the zones run through the hands, if you cover the whole of the front and/or back of the hand this will have a positive effect on the whole body. You can grip the comb in your fist so that the teeth dig into the palm of your hand, hold this for as long as feels comfortable, then move it slightly so that you do not damage the skin and apply pressure again. You can do this with each hand for a few minutes. The other way is to hold the comb in one hand and press it into the palm of the other, again holding the pressure in one area for as long as you can without experiencing too much discomfort then moving the comb and pressing again, trying to cover a large area of the palm. Don't press too hard on the back of the hand as this will hurt! The trick for dealing with discomfort is to relax into it, just accept it, try to keep your body relaxed, and it will lessen. You can use a brush in a similar way to a comb, and if the teeth have a blunt end you can apply a little more pressure. A brush with blunt teeth can be used in a rubbing motion (sharp teeth may scratch the skin); doing this gently on the back of each hand can be a great way to stimulate the healing reflexes in all the zones and relax the nervous system.

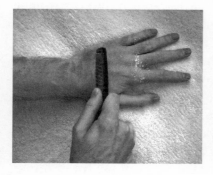 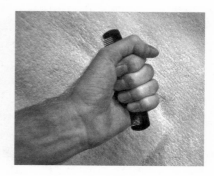

Finally it is worth investigating your own body with zone therapy. If you have a particular problem that you would like to treat, work out which of the 10 zones it might be in and then apply pressure to that zone in the hands or the feet or any other part of the body in that zone. Do this for a few minutes two or three times a day, continue for one week and see what happens! If you get great results continue the treatment on a less regular basis and if you get a complete cure stop the treatment one week from the time of complete recovery.

Some people believe that the central zone is the most important to treat on a regular basis. The central channel of the human life force energy system and the chakras run up the center of the body, and all the other meridians or channels branch off from this. Also, Buddhism explains that the root or very subtle mind is located at the level of the heart in the center of the body. If our central zone is strong and healthy the rest of the body will naturally follow.

One great way to treat the central zone is to bite your tongue! We start by sticking our tongue out as far as possible then we squeeze it between our teeth. Keep the tongue completely relaxed and apply pressure without causing yourself pain, after holding this for a few seconds you might be able to increase the pressure slightly, hold the same position for about 10 or 20 seconds. If you feel you are applying too much pressure release it immediately as the tongue is a delicate, complex, and essential piece of our body and much more sensitive than the hands and fingers, so we must not damage it in any way. Once released, draw your tongue in slightly and apply pressure again to the new area. Continue like this until you reach the tip of the tongue. You can also gently apply pressure on each side of the tongue with the teeth at the side of your mouth. At the end of this treatment your tongue should tingle but not be bruised or painful.

It is very important not to use this technique while walking or driving or working in any way. You must be sitting down and relaxed for it to be both safe and effective. You can do it at the same time as using the rubber band technique for example. Another complementary aid to this technique is to place both your palms over some part of the central area of your body like the solar plexus, navel, or at the level of your heart. This helps to channel healing energy into your body.

Just a note with respect to children: you can use all the above techniques gently but perhaps not the tongue-biting technique, especially with young children as they may forget and use it in an unsafe way or teach it to their friends. The other important point is to be very gentle with all the techniques and cause no discomfort or pain, as what might be slightly uncomfortable for an adult can be painful for a child.

7

Good practice

The main objective of reflexology is to restore health to body and mind as quickly and easily as possible. It would be wonderful if that were to happen every time reflexology is used. However, we do not live in a perfect world so the aims of reflexology have to be realistically adjusted to reflect what can be practically achieved with each individual patient. Sometimes we may only achieve a reduction in the severity of the symptoms and this improvement might have to be maintained with regular treatments. However, we can regard such a treatment to be successful if the patient is happy with such improvements. The patient's attitude to her or his condition is of paramount importance. This is where reflexology can have the most profound effects. Encouraging positive mental and emotional qualities through the treatment, listening, and sometimes giving good advice are some of the best ways you can help them. A positive mind is a wonderful "byproduct" of receiving reflexology and one of the most important factors in the healing process. We can even verify the power of a positive mind on health through the results of scientific research. It's official – being happy is good for you!

In fact, restoring a good mental attitude should be your number one priority. We will look at the reasons for this later but for now we can definitely say that a happy mind is a very useful thing! There are many people in this world who have to deal with severe suffering of one form or another yet many do so with a happy mind, a contented mind, a mind that wishes no more than that very happiness. Are such people healthy, do they need healing?

If you are embarking on a journey toward an understanding of the "way of healing" then from the start you need to develop a little wisdom to temper and shape the power of your compassionate wish to help others. Wisdom is essential. You can be the most technically accomplished and compassionate healer but without a little simple wisdom many of your actions can be misguided and your time and effort wasted. Strange as it may seem, good physical health might not always be the healer's main ambition. We will examine this later when we look at the cause and cure of disease and the nature of the mind.

Professional practice

If you wish to practice professionally, you will need to pursue a recognized course of study and obtain the relevant qualifications. This is as much for your own benefit as for the people you will be treating. You will need to obtain professional indemnity insurance and again you will need a recognized qualification for this. There are many reflexology courses available today as it is such a well-respected and widely known form of complementary therapy. Many of the people who study courses in reflexology and other complementary therapies have no intention of practicing professionally but simply wish to be able to treat friends and family. The courses are not difficult and are generally very interesting, enjoyable, and well structured so that anyone can complete them with confidence in their ability to treat others. You will also meet many people of like mind and benefit from the company and sharing of ideas about your chosen therapy.

You can start practicing the basic techniques straight away. You can do no damage and the more "hands-on" experience you get the better you will become, although again you should only practice on those you know well and never make any claims that you can cure any kind of illness. When friends and family experience the pleasure and positive results of a good treatment then you will have a long queue of willing patients beating a path to your door! Learning reflexology can be great fun and when you begin to get good results this can really encourage you to learn more and really hone your skills to perfection. There is a real sense of accomplishment and satisfaction in seeing the benefits others derive from your skills.

Preparing for treatment

If you are treating someone for the first time, put yourself in their position: how did you feel when you first received reflexology? Try to make them as welcome and comfortable as possible, without being over-bearing. Give them time to explain why they have come to see you and what they hope to gain from the treatment, i.e. their "intentions." Give yourself a suitable period of uninterrupted time; a full treatment usually lasts between 45 and 50 minutes depending on your experience and the patient's requirements. Try to avoid potential distractions by using an answer phone, not answering the front door, and asking others not to disturb you during the treatment. It can also be useful to have a clock within view to keep track of time. Some people are physically and mentally energized by reflexology and others are left feeling relaxed and ready to unwind, so be aware of this and don't take either as a good or a bad sign because the good results of a treatment can take days to become apparent. You will need a quiet, warm, peaceful, and clean environment in which to work. Of course if you are working from other people's homes you will have to make do and adapt accordingly. However, you can warn them beforehand that the treatment will be more effective if the room that you use is at least warm and quiet and that you will need not to be disturbed.

If you have access to a treatment room there are lots of things you can do to make it feel really peaceful and welcoming. Some obvious pointers are the décor: subtle colors and pleasant pictures are effective along with flowers, plants, and one or two comfy chairs to be used when you are talking to the client before and after the treatment. Also crystals, aromatherapy burners, and appropriate relaxing music all go to create the right conditions conducive to successful treatments. However, despite the best preparations if we do not know how to treat our client or patient with respect, empathy, wisdom, and understanding then we are fighting a losing battle. If the patient has confidence and faith in your abilities and feels relaxed and able to talk freely without fear of judgment then you can be assured that the barriers to healing will be gradually worn down.

Patient comfort

From the patient's point of view they need to be physically and mentally relaxed to receive the greatest benefit from the treatment. They will normally be lying down or sitting up with their arms on cushions on side tables, so that both arms can be fully relaxed and completely limp. Or you can just use one side table and let the other hand rest in the patient's lap. The hands need to be kept warm at all times. So as soon as the client has settled into a comfortable position place a small towel over both hands. When you are ready to begin the treatment simply unwrap the hand you are going to treat first.

The therapist also has to be as comfortable as possible during the session, especially if they intend to do several successive treatments. A chair that supports the lower back is essential and an erect but not stiff posture should be adopted so that your spine is not bent. Your back muscles will gradually strengthen with each treatment and this will prevent wear and tear on the spine. It is also useful if the chair is on wheels, like an office chair, and preferably without arms. This enables you to move around the patient because you may want to treat the hands sometimes from the front and sometimes from the back. A small table, perhaps also on wheels, is useful to keep those things that you need close at hand.

You will need to wash your hands before every treatment and possibly also the patient's hands. For the patient you could use some sort of antiseptic wipe but check first for any cuts or sensitive areas that might sting from using this. Of course, if you are using a damp cloth you will need a small bowl with warm water and some kind of antiseptic detergent diluted in it. If your hands are cold, warm them before starting the treatment. Cold hands can be a shock and hinder relaxation. You can warm your hands simply by clenching your fists tight then relaxing and shaking your hands; do this several times until the blood begins to flow. Alternatively you can put your hands in warm water for a few minutes then repeat the clenching exercise.

Always check the hands thoroughly before any treatment, especially the first. There are some skin conditions where it would be wiser not to treat the patient unless you use thin, medical grade, rubber gloves. This isn't ideal but if someone has a stubborn or persistent skin problem that you want to avoid contact with it is the only way to treat them. You definitely need a good knowledge of these before you treat people that you don't know well. If you intend to pursue a college course in reflexology then this is something that will be covered in detail.

First treatment

You may need to explain exactly what reflexology is, how it works, and what the treatment entails, so think about how you will do this. There is no reason to overload people with details but it can be helpful to explain the basics and it gives people confidence in your abilities if you obviously know what you are talking about. Also on the first treatment you will have to ask the person you are treating to read and sign a disclaimer. However, this is really only important if you are practicing reflexology professionally and being paid for your services. Such topics will be covered on a practitioners' training course, together with taking case notes and the client's personal details and medical history.

So if you are treating someone for the first time it may be helpful to tell them what to expect during a treatment. However, judge every situation as you think best; sometimes it may not seem appropriate as the patient may then be thinking about what might happen instead of just relaxing. Here are some examples of what you may wish to tell them, if it feels like the right thing to do:

- How long the treatment takes, and that the treatment is done solely on the hands using just your own hands
- Demonstrate the basic hand techniques and let them know that they can just relax and switch off
- They may experience warmth in and around the body and/or coming from your hands, occasionally it may feel cool instead!
- Also tingling sensations may be felt in and around the body
- A sense of heaviness or lightness
- They may feel very relaxed or even sleepy, it's fine to fall asleep
- They may want to talk, which is fine
- Their body may sweat slightly or twitch sometimes and they may feel some "movement" within the body as they relax
- Their stomach may "gurgle" as their body relaxes.
- Also their throat may become dry, so have a glass of water at hand, and tissues for a "runny" nose!

Explain that these are all natural reactions. Some people may have much deeper and more profound experiences and/or emotional releases, so again a box of tissues and of course an ability to listen may be useful. Try to be open and accept whatever arises and trust that the client will know consciously or subconsciously what they are ready to release and/or deal with. The more genuine trust and confidence you have in others' natural healing abilities the easier it will be for those qualities to naturally arise within them. From the practitioner's side, developing this trust in the process of natural healing is part of our own healing and growth, it also creates the right atmosphere and conditions conducive to "ripening" the client's own self-healing potential.

It is important to have a relaxed state of mind and to enjoy your work. There is not much point in treating others when we have a negative, impatient, bored, or inattentive attitude. It will show in your work, and people will notice and lose confidence in you and the treatment. In fact, if we can strive to develop a relaxed, peaceful, and compassionate state of mind then this will greatly assist the effectiveness of the treatment. We may think that this is impossible: how can a state of mind positively affect an apparently physical therapy? Well we can look at this in different ways. Certainly if we went to see a therapist who had an impatient and condescending attitude this would make us feel uncomfortable and, alternatively, when we are in the company of people who are deeply peaceful and caring we naturally feel some benefits from their presence. Also, many people believe that the healer is acting as a channel for healing energy and that reflexology can act as a kind of energetic gateway for the patient to receive this. Some people definitely have a natural ability to heal others simply through touch and it is often those who are attracted to the healing professions that possess such latent healing potential. To successfully channel such healing energy, wherever you believe it comes from, you need a peaceful, relaxed mind, a feeling of compassion or empathy for your patient, and a wish for them to receive whatever they need without grasping at success or being worried about failure in this regard. If you have a religion then faith is very important and you can always say silent prayers for your patient before each treatment and ask for guidance, blessings, and healing inspiration. If you do not see regular miracles you should not be surprised, disappointed, or discouraged. You do not know what people really need in their lives. It is difficult for you to see the "big picture" and sometimes there is a lot to be gained from having to develop the inner resources to live with a challenging illness. If you can impart this information skillfully and at the right time then you may be doing your client a greater favor than if you were to simply take away their illness or disability.

Give the patient time to talk and collect themselves after the treatment and have a drink and a biscuit handy as a little sugar and liquid can help people become "grounded" and alert after a very relaxing treatment. This is especially important if they have to drive home. If you are doing several successive treatments give yourself a few minutes' rest between each treatment and set a mental intention to relax and recharge yourself. Don't take on too much too soon. In the beginning just do a few treatments per week. This will give you time to build up your strength, stamina, and concentration. If you find that you are drained after a treatment, are you too tense during the treatment or are you using too much pressure? A gentle touch is usually all that is required. We are not forcing the patient to get better, just gently encouraging good health to arise.

How many treatments?

Usually a full treatment once a week is more than adequate. We may do this for six to eight weeks and then reduce it to every two weeks and then once a month until a complete cure is established. We can usually tell after the first three or four treatments if the condition we are treating is going to respond favorably to reflexology. In more serious and long-term cases once a week is usually enough but it is really up to the patient to decide how long they wish to continue regular treatment. Occasionally, when people are very ill, two gentle half-hour treatments per week are more pleasant, relaxing, and less demanding on the body's abilities to expel the toxins that are being released. Also over-stimulating a body's healing system that is already overtaxed with a serious illness can cause more problems. The answer is "gently does it." Some people may not need any follow-up treatments after the initial six or eight and some people may just want to come for perhaps three treatments as a form of seasonal detox and revitalizing treatment. So we are not only there to help cure and relieve sickness and disease but also to act as a form of life-enhancing and revitalizing therapist.

Some people may find other complementary therapies to be more appropriate for them. Of course most complementary therapies are complementary! So the patient could be using two or three therapies at the same time without adverse effects. The only thing we need to be wary of is that the body needs time to recover from detoxification and too much treatment can make the patient feel ill while detox is occurring. In this regard the more severe the illness the gentler and more patient we must be with the patient!

When treating children their attention span and hence their ability to lie still for a full treatment may be limited. So we can either give them shorter, more frequent treatments or treat them when they are asleep, or sitting in their parent's lap. Obviously if we do not know the child well a parent or guardian must be present throughout the treatment. It's not surprising that children are usually more naturally understanding and intuitively wise to natural healing techniques, consequently this trust and openness often brings swifter results.

Typical reactions

Typical reactions during and after a reflexology treatment are:

- increased energy
- inner peace and a feeling of warmth within and/or around the body

- gentle tingling sensations, especially in the hands which may also feel hot
- a sense of energy flowing in and/or around the body
- clearer senses
- lessening of stress and emotional problems
- improved physical health
- increased ability to deal positively with stressful situations
- increased clarity of mind and deeper intuitive or inner wisdom
- a sense of "coming home" and of being in touch with "the flow" of life
- deepening of spiritual awareness and experiences, e.g. seeing or sensing auras, energy, colors etc.
- a general feeling of being more whole, healthy and happy, a more complete sense of self.

Everyone is different, and some people may feel nothing during a treatment and this is also normal! Reflexology works in the way that we need it as individuals so we should not expect any two people to react in the same way, even when they have the same illness.

Occasionally a "cleansing" period of body and mind may occur after the first few reflexology treatments; this might be especially true if the patient has a serious illness. This might involve:

- a short minor illness, i.e. cold, flu
- sweating
- headaches
- frequent urination
- a need to sleep more
- a need to drink more
- temporary loss or increase in appetite
- some other minor physical problems, some type of emotional release i.e. crying, laughing.

These symptoms are a positive sign that the patient's body is working well to heal itself and we can encourage the client by telling them this. However, it is not a definite sign that they will regain health so always be careful what you say. If symptoms of detox are persistent and severe, reduce the regularity of treatments and the length of treatment or use a gentler touch. Encouraging the patient to drink plenty of clean water, perhaps even three or four pints a day, can also help.

It is quite common for people to feel tired or sleepy for days after a treatment. This is a good sign that they are beginning to learn how to finally "open" and fully relax. Often the amount of stress we carry goes unnoticed as we move from one thing in life to another. The habit of stress and the layers of stress gradually accumulate in our system, both physically and mentally, to the extent that we never allow ourselves time to just "be" who we are. We can even build up and carry stress with us from one lifetime to another for many lifetimes. This accumulated stress acts as a barrier to healing, inner peace, and a sense of our timeless spirituality, to the extent that we forget our true nature as primarily spiritual beings. Practicing natural healing techniques, meditation, prayer, or deep relaxation is a way to gradually release stress, cleanse the body and mind, and re-introduce us to ourselves!

Learning to deeply relax, open our mind, and allow stress, often in the form of negative thought patterns, to arise from within and fall away can sometimes be unnerving, as we often feel these aspects of our mind are part of our own sense of self or true identity. So this process can sometimes leave us feeling a little "naked" and unsure of ourselves. However, given time and a little positive experience we will develop the confidence and wish to consciously seek and appreciate this inner path toward a more whole and healthy way of living and being.

Helping the healing process

There are some things that we can do to help the natural healing process. They are not essential and not everyone would find them helpful, so only suggest them to patients if you think they are appropriate.

- Eat healthily, with a well-balanced diet including lots of fresh fruit and vegetables
- Cut down on alcohol
- Cut down on smoking or stop altogether if you can
- Avoid caffeine drinks and try to drink lots of still mineral water or herbal teas
- Cut down on chocolate, sweets, or other refined foods
- Try to eat only fresh food products and perhaps consider a short water or juice fast, but only if you have experience of fasting
- Avoid confrontational or stressful situations, try to keep a peaceful, happy and relaxed mind
- Spend some quiet time on your own in a peaceful place, go for walks in pleasant surroundings
- Meditate or pray for 10-20 minutes each day or simply spend this time in silence or reading a spiritual text
- Think positively! Essentially try to approach life with a relaxed, positive and open mind.

The effects of following these simple guidelines can be quite dramatic. If we ask our patients to set a target to follow them all for seven days, or even better three weeks, they will see that it makes a big difference to their state of well-being. These physical and mental benefits can really inspire them to continue for longer periods until they become regular habits. They are sowing the seeds for good health now and in the future.

If you think there may be a serious undetected physical problem try not to alarm your client but do encourage them to see their own doctor, especially if they also feel something is "not right." They can always ask and should never be afraid to see another doctor for a second opinion about their current medical condition. If you are a professional complementary therapist all your clients who are seeking help for serious medical complaints should come to you after or while they are being treated by their own doctor.

Becoming a good healer

On the surface it appears that reflexology is just a physical therapy but it is much more than this. The client/therapist relationship is of paramount importance. Obviously any patient would be put off by an overbearing, self-important, and "loud" therapist. These qualities would leave the patient in doubt about the ability of the practitioner and the effectiveness of the therapy. Conversely if the reflexologist is quietly confident, kind, considerate, patient, and willing to listen then this immediately instills confidence and a certain amount of faith and encouragement in the patient. As therapists we need to be in a frame of mind that allows the patient to feel comfortable and at ease with us. Really we need to be at a place in our own mental and spiritual evolution where we have developed certain qualities that allow us to be a catalyst for healing.

This may sound a little mystical but it is a truth. If we are shallow, materialistic, self-centered, and in it for the money, praise, or recognition of others then we really have nothing to give. How do we develop the special qualities that will transform us in to an effective therapist? We really have to work this out for ourselves. However, the first step is simply to develop the wish to be such a person and much of the rest is simply learning from our life experiences and interpreting them with wisdom. Some people find following a recognized path of spiritual and personal growth to be very helpful.

In everyday life we meet some people that we feel "uncomfortable" with and some that we just don't like! If you are faced with this situation with a reflexology client, not liking them will not affect the quality of the physical treatment but will obviously affect the quality of the client/therapist relationship. In these situations try to be like a good doctor and develop a warm and friendly professional relationship equally with all your "patients," without being particularly attached to some or averse to others. Another strategy is to use the situation to discover more about yourself. Think "why do I not like this person, what is this situation telling me about myself?" Often the people and situations that we find difficult to deal with are reflections of some part of our own mind that we do not fully "own" or understand, like a missing piece of the jigsaw.

This also applies to situations or people we are deeply attached to or depend upon for our happiness and peace of mind. Most of our relationships are tainted with aspects of "need" or aversion; often we need the approval or simply the presence of others to feel secure, happy, and whole and it easy to think of many things we dislike or disapprove of in others. We don't have to be completely self-sufficient and separate or completely reliant on others for our well-being, there is a middle way. We can learn to give and receive without needing others to feel whole or pushing others away to feel "free." This way of living leads to meaningful relationships and a sense of personal freedom. This feeling of equanimity is also a good attribute to develop and apply to all areas of our lives. If we try to cultivate a balanced, warm, and friendly attitude toward everyone we meet all our relationships will be naturally harmonious.

On the whole, given the right conditions, everyone has the natural ability to heal themselves. In some ways being a reflexologist gives us the ability to provide these healing conditions, when others cannot initially help themselves. The less we interfere with this process the better. Too much well-intentioned advice can confuse people who may already be trying to deal with a difficult illness and changes in lifestyle. We don't always know what is best for others! Often we want to give what others do not need and trying to provide answers for others can definitely lessen their ability to resolve their own issues.

The "good" healer to some extent steps back from being a "solver of problems" and becomes more of an "enabler" or simply a healing witness. This allows people to draw through the healer, and from within themselves, what they actually need to help them overcome or transform their own situation – physically, mentally, or emotionally. This "sustainable healing" allows people to develop the qualities that either consciously or subconsciously they need to help themselves. It also provides them with the skills they may need to deal with similar problems in the future. This can be a slow process at first, but gradually healing the inner problems lays the foundations for a deep and lasting overall healing that is more than worth a little extra time and effort.

If you seem to be attracting people with similar problems this is an indication that you may need to move forward in those areas as well: there is usually a strong connection between the problems people bring to healers and their own "issues." You can't expect other people to change for the better if you are not prepared to be honest about and challenge your own shortcomings! You don't have to be perfect, just prepared to learn more about yourself. Try not to feel pride about being a healer or act in a superior way; this can be a real barrier to your own healing and to improving your own healing abilities. If you try to be honest about your weaknesses, without being hard on yourself and if you are able to share your problems and ask for help when you need it, then your own ability to heal yourself and others will continue to grow.

Realistic expectations

All illness has its root cause in the mind and therein also lies the cure of all illness. If the mind is not ready or willing to change on an obvious or subtle level, the illness will not be cured, or we may only achieve temporary relief. It appears that everyone has the wish to be healthy; however, very few people know themselves well enough to recognize that their illness is an expression of some part of their own mind that does not wish to be healthy or that does not know how to be well. We can re-teach ourselves to be well if we are willing to be patient and look within for the answers and not hand over the responsibility for our health to others. Healing works on all levels but principally on a mental and emotional level first, so don't be surprised if a physical condition does not disappear overnight. Good reflexology works to achieve long-term improvements by helping the person address, heal, and release the issues that initially caused the problem and this may happen obviously or in a very subtle way. Sometimes just learning to accept and live with a major illness is all we can help people achieve, depending on the severity and duration of the problem. We should never regard this as failure; if their quality of life has improved only a little we should be pleased with this progress.

Good intentions

To make our healing actions more powerful and meaningful there are two simple ideas we can adapt from the Buddhist way of life. If we are preparing to practice reflexology, whether on ourselves or others, we can begin with a short prayer, affirmation, or mental "intention" and finish with a brief "dedication." Intention is everything! Our intention is what creates our "karma." Although this is explained in more detail later, briefly, everything we do, say, and think, every action of body, speech, and mind, creates a potential in the mind for a corresponding physical, verbal, or mental reaction in the future. It also creates the habit or tendency for us to repeat such actions in the future and an increased wish or compulsion to keep performing similar negative actions. If we perform negative actions we can expect negative re-actions sooner or later.

Also if we generally have a negative approach to life we are more likely to create the conditions that attract problems and difficult circumstances. Likewise the positive energy we create by developing patience or kindness or giving a reflexology treatment will return to us as a very positive experience in one form or another. If we set a very positive mental intention before we perform any type of healing action, including reflexology, or indeed any form of giving or beneficial action, then this will greatly increase the power of our karma. If this intention is wise and heartfelt the consequences of our actions can benefit countless living beings, although we cannot directly see this incredible result. Basically, if our motivation is to benefit others rather than ourselves then this will create very powerful and positive karma. To set an intention we just need to sit quietly for a few minutes, calm the mind, and think of those people we would like to benefit. Then we can simply think or pray:

> *Through the force of these healing actions may (name the people you are thinking of) find lasting happiness and good health.*

Or even more powerfully:

> *May all living beings gain lasting benefit from these healing actions.*

When the treatment is over we can dedicate our positive actions or good karma. Dedication is similar to intention. If we consciously "dedicate" or direct this positive energy for a specific purpose, this can be a very powerful way of manifesting our intentions, achieving our goals, and accelerating our spiritual or personal growth. Whenever we create positive energy by helping others in any way or by consciously developing positive states of mind, we can dedicate this energy.

Choosing a purpose or direction for dedication is similar to creating an intention. If we can choose a purpose that will benefit many people then this wish will be fulfilled more easily than a purely selfish purpose. To dedicate after any positive action we can simply think or pray:

> *May this positive energy be fully dedicated for the greatest good of all living beings.*

or

> *May every living being benefit from these positive actions.*

Perhaps the greatest goals we could wish for are:

> *Through the force of this positive energy may every living being be released from suffering and may we all find true lasting happiness swiftly and easily.*

and/or

> *Through the force of these positive actions may my wisdom and compassion continually increase for the benefit of others.*

This mental practice only takes a short time but this small gesture is a very special practice. We can easily waste or destroy the potential of previous positive actions or good karma simply by developing negative states of mind like anger, guilt, or jealousy. *Sincere* and heartfelt dedication is like "banking" or protecting the potential of our positive actions for our own and others' future benefit. In this way the potential of our good thoughts, words, and deeds can only increase and will produce excellent results for ourselves and everyone in the future.

8

Traditional Chinese medicine

Reflexology is rooted in Chinese medicine. This fascinating holistic system of healing has diagnosed, treated, and prevented illness for at least 3000 years. You do not need to have an understanding of Chinese medicine to be a good reflexologist but it can help you to develop a more holistic understanding of your therapy. The information in this chapter is provided by www.aworldofchinesemedicine.com. It is recommended that the reader seek appropriate training before applying any of this knowledge in practice.

Chinese medicine is based on the principles of internal balance and harmony. This highly refined and complex discipline works to regenerate the body's organs and systems. Each human is viewed as a mini-ecosystem that shares common traits with the earth on which we live.

The Chinese have a concept of vital energy known as chi or qi (pronounced chee), which is the basis of all life. In the body, chi is transported via the 12 major energetic pathways known as meridians. Although these meridians cannot be seen with the naked eye, modern science has proven their existence through electronic detection. Each meridian connects to one of the major organs, and chi is said to power the organ, enabling effective functioning. For example, the path of the heart meridian travels from the heart, to the armpit, and down the inside of the arm to the little finger. This explains why some individuals with heart conditions will express a tingling feeling running down the arm and into the fingers. Chi is regulated by the interdependent forces of Yin and Yang.

The Chinese symbol for Yin literally means "the dark side of the mountain," and represents the qualities of cold, still, dark, below, weakness, and void. The Chinese symbol for Yang translates to "the sunny side of the mountain," and therefore represents the opposite qualities of Yin: heat, activity, light, above, strength, and solidity. A person's constitution, or the nature of the disease, is determined by the aspects of Yin and Yang. Harmony and balance of this union yields a healthy state, whereas excess or deficiency of either Yin or Yang is thought to lead to illness.

The basic principles of this complete medical system can be explained in seven sections:

- Causes of Disharmony
- Meridians
- Five Elements
- Vital Substances
- Yin and Yang
- Zangfu
- Diagnosis

1. Causes of Disharmony

Traditional Chinese Medicine views the cause of disease in three main areas: external causes, internal causes, and a group of miscellaneous causes, which primarily involve lifestyle.

THE SIX EXTERNAL CAUSES

The six external causes of disease, also known as the six evils, are causes of disharmony that relate to climatic conditions. Just as extremes of wind, cold, heat, dampness, dryness, and summer heat can have devastating effects on the world in which we live, they can also seriously alter the balance within the body by diminishing, or blocking the flow of chi in the organs.

Wind is the most prevalent of the six external factors, and refers to the ability of an illness to spread within the body. Symptoms commonly linked with wind include chills, fever, colds, flu, nasal congestion, headaches, allergies, arthritic and rheumatic conditions, as well as dizziness and vertigo.

Cold-related imbalances manifest as conditions that diminish the body's immune system, such as colds, cough, upper respiratory allergies, as well as poor circulation, anemia, and weak digestion.

Heat conditions are described as hot and inflammatory, exacerbated by hot weather and exposure to direct heat. They represent an over-active metabolic process, which can result in hypertension, hyperthyroid, ulcers, colitis, and inflamed arthritic joints, as well as flu and skin rashes.

Dampness symptoms are created through the intake of oily and fluidic foods, as well as wet weather. These symptoms may include swelling, obesity, the formation of cysts, tumors, and lumps, and an increased production of phlegm. This phlegm production can affect the sinuses and upper respiratory passages, including the lungs and bronchioles.

Dryness can damage vegetation, and creates similar imbalances within the body, causing disorders of the lungs, sinuses, large intestine, skin, digestion, and reproductive organs.

Summer heat, or an overexposure to sunlight and hot weather, can yield conditions such as heat stroke, dizziness, nausea, extreme thirst, and exhaustion.

THE SEVEN INTERNAL CAUSES

The seven internal causes, otherwise known as the Seven Emotions, are illnesses brought about by intense, prolonged, or suppressed feelings, and are defined as follows:

Sadness decreases the flow of chi in the lungs and heart, and is associated with depression, fatigue, shortness of breath, asthma, allergies, cold, and flu.

Grief is similar to sadness, and injures the lungs, decreases immunity to colds and flu, and is associated with chronic upper respiratory diseases such as emphysema, allergies, and asthma.

Pensiveness, or over-engaging the mind in activities such as worry, thought, or study can deplete spleen chi, and may result in edema, digestive disorders, low appetite, and fatigue.

Fear, or paranoia causes chi to descend, resulting in potential harm to the kidneys, lower back, or joints when this emotion is ever present.

Fright, or shock, is unlike fear in the sense that the onset is very sudden, causing one's chi to diverge. The rapid change in flow first affects the heart in symptoms such as breathlessness and palpitations, then moves to the lower body in a similar fashion to fear, damaging the kidneys, lower back, and joints.

Anger encompasses all the negative emotions of rage, irritability, frustration, and resentment, and causes the chi to rise inappropriately. Anger is associated with headaches, mental confusion, dizziness, and hypertension.

Joy in Chinese medicine refers to excess, or overabundance, and relates to illness relative to overindulgence. Damage to the heart may result, and the conditions of hysteria, muddled thought, and insomnia may arise.

2. The meridian system

In addition to chi (qi), traditional Chinese medicine recognizes a subtle energy system by which chi is circulated through the body. This transportation system is referred to as the channels or meridians. There are 12 main meridians in the body, six yin and six yang, and each relates to one of the Zangfu, or organs.

To better visualize the concept of chi, and the meridians, think of the meridians as a riverbed, over which water flows and irrigates the land: feeding, nourishing, and sustaining the substance through which it flows. (In western medicine, the concept would be likened to the blood flowing through the circulatory system.) If a dam were placed at any point along the river, the nourishing effect that the water had on the whole river would stop at the point the dam was placed.

The same is true in relation to chi and the meridians. When chi becomes blocked, the rest of the body that was being nourished by the continuous flow now suffers. Illness and disease can result if the flow is not restored. Acupuncture is one tool used to restore the flow of chi, by inserting needles into the acupuncture points (located on the meridians). These insertions are said to clear any residing blockages, or dams, thus freeing the river to better feed the body in its entirety.

3. The five elements in Chinese medicine

The five elements, also called "Wu Xing," represent the processes that are fundamental to the cycles of nature, and therefore correspond to the human body. In relation to the five elements, the cycle of processes can be represented as:

- wood feeds fire
- fire creates ashes which form earth
- inside the earth, metal which is heated liquefies and produces water vapor
- water generated then nourishes the trees, or wood

The five elements, their characteristics, and their inter-relationships with the body can be defined as:

Fire: Hot, ascending, light, and energy as embodied in the traditional Chinese medicine (TCM) functions of the heart (yin) and small intestine (yang). The fire element also affects the complementary organ processes of the pericardium (yin) and the triple warmer, which is representative of the upper, lower, and middle parts of the body, as well as the circulation of fluids in these areas (yang). Joy (overindulgence) is the emotion, which creates imbalance within this element.

Earth: Productive, fertile, growth. The earth element relates to the stomach (yang) and the spleen (yin). The stomach begins the process of digestive breakdown, while the spleen transforms and transports the energy from food and drink throughout the body. Pensiveness is the emotion, which creates imbalance within this element.

Metal: As a conductor, this element includes the lungs (yin), which move vital energy throughout the body, and the large intestine (yang), which is responsible for receiving and discharging waste. Sadness, or grieving is the emotion, which creates imbalance within this element.

Water: Wet, descending, flowing. The water element represents the urinary bladder (yang), and the kidney (yin). The bladder receives, stores, and excretes urine. Water metabolism dissipates fluids throughout the body, moistening it, then accumulating in the kidneys. The kidneys also store the essence, and serve as the root of yin and yang for the entire body. Fear and paranoia are the emotions, which create imbalance within this element.

Wood: Strong, rooted. The wood element represents the liver (yin), and the gall bladder (yang). The liver stores blood, and regulates the smooth flow of chi. The gall bladder is responsible for storing and excreting bile. Anger is the emotion that creates imbalance within the liver, while indecisiveness is relative to the gall bladder.

4. Vital substances

Traditional Chinese medicine views the human body as a mini eco-system, which therefore shares the same qualities as nature. Just as the earth contains air, water, and land, the basic substances of the human body are chi, body fluids, blood, and essence.

Chi is the vital energy that gives us our capacity to move, think, and feel. It protects from illness, and warms the body. Chi is derived from two main sources: the air we breathe and the food we eat. When the supply of chi to the body is depleted or blocked, organ function is adversely affected by the inability to transform and transport the "energy" necessary to fight illness and disease.

Body fluids (called Jin Ye) are the liquids that protect, nurture, and lubricate the body in conjunction with the blood. The moisture nourishes the skin, muscles, joints, spine, bone marrow, and brain. Dehydration results in conditions such as dry skin and constipation, while excess fluids manifest in symptoms such as lethargy, and increased production of phlegm.

Blood is the material foundation for bone, nerve, skin, muscle, and organ creation. It also contains the Shen (spirit), which balances the psyche.

Essence, or Jing, is the body's reproductive and regenerative substance. Essence regulates growth, development, and reproduction, and promotes and works with chi to help protect the body from external factors.

The vital substances circulate through the pathways, or meridians, linking all parts of the body. When flowing smoothly they contribute to the healthy state, but if these substances are congested or depleted, symptoms as varied as aches, tension, swelling, asthma, indigestion, and fatigue may result from the disruption.

5. Yin and yang

In Chinese medicine, health is represented as a balance of yin and yang. These two forces represent the bipolar manifestation of all things in nature, and because of this, one must be present to allow the other to exist. Hence, where there is above there is below, whatever has a front also has a back, night is followed by day, etc. On an emotional level, one would not know joy had one never experienced pain.

It is important to note that the balance of yin and yang is not always exact, even when the body is healthy. Under normal circumstances the balance is in a state of constant change, based on both the external and internal environment.

For example, during times of anger, a person's mood is more fiery, or yang, and yet once the anger has subsided, and a quiet peaceful state is achieved, yin may dominate.

This shift in the balance of yin and yang is very natural. It is when the balance is consistently altered, and one (be it yin or yang) regularly dominates the other, that health is compromised, resulting in illness and disease.

Traditional Chinese medicine practitioners attempt to determine the exact nature of the imbalance, and then correct it through the use of acupuncture, herbal remedies, exercise, diet, and lifestyle. As balance is restored in the body, so is health.

6. Zangfu

Zangfu is the term used to describe various yin and yang organs in the body. A yin organ is called a Zang, while a yang organ is called a Fu. Although the organs are identified by their western anatomical names, traditional Chinese medicine views their function on a far broader scope, due in part to the concepts of chi and essence, their flow, and storage responsibilities.

The 12 organs of Chinese medicine, which correspond to the 12 meridians, or channels within the body, are classified according to the functions of transformation (yin organs), or transportation (yang organs). The Zang is made up of the six solid (yin) organs: the heart, pericardium (sac surrounding the heart), lungs, spleen, liver, and kidney. The Fu consists of the six hollow (yang) organs: the small intestine, triple warmer (an organ function), stomach, large intestine, gall bladder, and the urinary bladder.

7. Traditional Chinese medicine diagnosis methods

The diagnostic process of Chinese medicine involves four areas, known as the Four Examinations. These are:

Observation of the patient's complexion, eyes, tongue, nails, gait (overall physical appearance), openness, and emotional demeanor.

Listening and smelling, the focus being on the sound of the voice and breathing, as well as any odors associated with the body, or breath.

Questioning for information on present and past complaints including appetite, digestion, bowel movement, bladder, sweat, pain, patterns of sleep, family health history, work, living habits, physical environment, and emotional life.

Palpation, or touching the body to determine temperature, moisture, pain, or sensitivity, and the taking of the pulse. The Chinese method of pulse taking involves placing three fingers on each wrist to measure a total of 12 pulses, each associated with a corresponding meridian. Fourteen different pulse characteristics (slow, rapid, full, empty, etc.) are compared with each of the 12 pulses, and are used to determine which organ is not working properly.

Treatments aim to adjust and restore the yin/yang balance, and may incorporate one or more therapies including acupuncture, herbal remedies, exercise and diet.

OBSERVATION

The observation portion of diagnosis begins the moment the patient appears before the practitioner. In this step, the practitioner is forming an initial impression of the patient, while assessing the seriousness of the condition based on four main considerations:

Vitality: the color, complexion, and luster of the skin, and the overall general impression of the patient are key points in observation. The appearance of the face is an excellent indicator of vitality as all the acupuncture meridians flow to the face, by their primary or secondary pathways, and the state of blood and chi is very evident in this area. In addition, the color of the face may reveal problems in the functioning of the organs. For example, black circles under the eyes could indicate kidney weakness, whereas red coloring (which relates to heat or fire) is linked with the heart. Black or blue coloring is linked with the kidneys, blue-green may involve the liver, and white implies a lung problem.

Body appearance: the appearance of the body can also provide the practitioner with good information as to where the problems lie. At this point the practitioner is mainly looking for the distribution of fat, type of build, appearance of body hair, etc. For example, it is difficult for yang chi to be distributed in a body with excess fat, therefore an overweight person is more susceptible to cardiac arrest and stoke.

Facial features: facial expressions tell the practitioner about the psychological status of the patient, whether it be sad, happy, anxious, or overjoyed, and are a point of consideration prior to making a diagnosis. The features themselves, including the eyes, nose, mouth, and lips, can also provide evidence of excess or deficient conditions causing imbalance in the body.

The tongue and its coating: the inspection of the tongue is a vital diagnostic procedure in the practice of traditional Chinese medicine. The color, coating, shape, and texture of various parts of the tongue yield information about the state of the organs. A normal tongue is moist and has an "appropriate" red color. A light red or pale tongue is a sign of deficiency in both chi and blood. A thick, purple-colored tongue is often associated with alcoholism, while cracks in the tongue show dryness, heat, and deficient yin. Prior to an examination, it is important not to eat or drink anything that will discolor the tongue and give a misleading impression to the practitioner.

LISTENING AND SMELLING

A significant aspect of this part of diagnosis is the breathing of the patient and the sound of the voice. A loud assertive voice suggests a yang pattern, while a weak or timid voice suggests the opposite, a yin pattern. Restless and heavy breathing occurs in an excess syndrome whereas shallow breathing is indicative of a deficient condition. Even the sound of a cough gives an indication of the level of phlegm in the lungs, and can be loud and sudden or weak and persistent.

The odor of the body and its excretions are also important aids in diagnosis, and require many years of experience to perfect. As such, this method is more widely practiced in traditional eastern diagnosis than it is in the western practices.

In general terms, there are two distinct smells, which are considered to differentiate between the presence of a hot, excess condition and a cold, deficient one. Yang (hot, excess) conditions are associated with a rancid or rotten smell and yin (cold, deficient) conditions possess a strong, fishy aroma. As a rule, any unusual or abnormal odors can indicate an illness, those listed above are merely a guideline.

QUESTIONING

During the first visit, a considerable amount of time is spent asking the patient for details about his or her general condition. These questions relate to all emotional, physical, and energy-related signs and symptoms, and can help the practitioner form a more complete picture of the patient's condition. A full medical history is usually taken, including details of past illness, operations, and physical and mental traumas. While these issues may not seem pertinent to the patient at this juncture, they do provide important insights into the pattern of disharmony existing within the patient.

Other important questions which may be asked are:

- Preferences for heat or cold
- Frequency and consistency of urination and defecation
- Sleep patterns
- Diet and thirst
- Menstrual cycle (length, pain associated, heaviness of bleeding, etc.)
- Headaches (when they occur, where and under what circumstances)
- Perspiration (amount, time of day, circumstances)

In addition, the practitioner may inquire regarding the nature of any pain or discomfort, as reactions to heat or cold may point to patterns of excess and deficiency, such as imbalances in yin and yang. For example, if pain is relieved by heat, a cold condition (yin) is indicated. If the reverse is true, such as a discomfort alleviated by cold, a yang condition could be present. The site(s) of the pain are also noted as they may indicate a blockage or stagnation of chi within the meridians of the body.

PALPATION

Palpation, or touching, is a form of diagnosis made by feeling and tapping local areas of the body to ascertain:

- Painful areas
- Temperature of the skin (heat, cold)
- Swelling
- Perspiration
- Color

Pulse diagnosis, as it applies to traditional Chinese medicine, is the most important form of palpation, and is very different from that of western physicians. In performing pulse palpation, the practitioner places the index, middle, and ring fingers on the radial artery. Three degrees of pressure, the light touch, the medium touch, and the heavy touch are applied to the region and correspond to the upper, middle, and lower areas of the body. In traditional terms, there are 28 pulse classifications, which describe the way the pulse feels to the fingertip. Some examples of these classifications are:

- **Slippery** – feels like a rolling pearl in a basin, very fluid and full
- **Choppy** – has no strength and is irregular
- **Full** – large and rounded, can be felt at all levels
- **Empty** – hard to detect or felt only slightly at the superficial level when pressure is applied
- **Slow** – slower than the normal rate of four to five beats per breath
- **Rapid** – six to seven beats per breath
- **Superficial** – easily felt on the skin surface
- **Deep** – only felt with a heavy touch

These, along with 20 other descriptions, must be taken into consideration during pulse diagnosis. This requires a tremendous amount of skill and practice, and when properly executed is one of the most important and accurate means of correctly diagnosing a patient. In fact, pulse and tongue diagnosis are considered to be the "two pillars" of the four examinations in traditional practice.

The information in this chapter has been kindly provided by www.aworldofchinesemedicine.com, an excellent resource site for anyone interested in this ancient and well-respected system of natural medicine.

9

Understanding sickness and health

The body and the mind cannot be separated in terms of understanding the cause and cure of ill-health. Conventional medicine has for a long time ignored this vital and important link, choosing to look at the health of the patient from a purely physical perspective. There is really no doubt that the body and mind have an intimate dependent relationship and that good physical health is closely related to good mental, emotional, and spiritual health.

Chinese and Tibetan medicine suggests that physical illness is directly related to the quality of our internal energies (chi/qi). As our mind is supported and greatly influenced by our internal energies we can say that the predominant negative state of mind that accompanies an illness can be regarded as a symptom of the negative internal energy that is creating the conditions for the illness to manifest. We cannot say that the negative state of mind is the *cause* of the illness, as many "New Age" thinkers believe. If this were true then everyone with a particular negative state of mind would develop the same illness or at least some illness. Also, everyone with a very positive state of mind would never be ill, but this is obviously not the case. We could say that, along with poor quality internal energies, negative minds are a "condition" that encourages illness to arise. However, as explained later we need to look deeper within the nature of the mind to discover the actual cause of illness.

Positive states of mind encourage and create healthy internal energies and vice versa. As physical health is directly related to the quality of our internal energies therefore it is also directly affected by our thoughts and emotions. We can prove this by simple logical reasoning. Some people can remain perfectly happy and content while experiencing poor health and even in the face of death, when the internal energies that create good health have become weak and impure. Plants and trees can also develop diseases and die, resulting from poor internal energies, and they have no mind or consciousness. So this shows that life force energy has a direct influence on health, but that the accompanying mind, although not a cause of illness, can have an influence on it by prolonging or shortening an illness or by influencing its severity. There is much evidence to support this; for example, we know that our immune system is directly affected by our state of mind and that people with long-term illness stand a much better chance of improving if they have a positive outlook. This mental influence is greatly increased if we can use our mind to consciously improve our internal energies through positive thinking and meditation.

What actually causes poor quality energy to arise and encourage illness will be examined later when we look at the laws of "karma," the root cause of all our problems and good fortune. The way in which the various internal energies or subtle winds, as they are called in Buddhism, affect and control physical and mental health is a very detailed area for study. There are Buddhist texts available that fully explain this fascinating subject (see Appendix 2); however, you do not need a detailed knowledge of this to be a good healer.

Opportunities for change

Illness often dispels pride and helps us develop such qualities as patience and contentment. Serious illness really concentrates the mind; it can certainly make us think more deeply about what we value in life and help us to reassess our priorities, our attitudes, and our lifestyle. Of course no one would recommend "learning from illness" as a path of choice, but there are so many examples of people whose lives have been positively transformed simply by learning to look at themselves and their lives in a new light. Buddha said, "illness has many good qualities"! This may seem like a strange philosophy for a therapist or healer to share with their clients when so many people prefer to view illness as something to fight against with all your energy. Unfortunately there are many instances when projecting too much energy at a problem by being "blindly" or unrealistically positive will just make things worse.

We have to strike a balance in our approach to health and illness. Be realistic but positive, deal with the day-to-day reality of being ill but don't rule out miracles. The people who learn to wisely adapt and learn to live with long-term illness are living examples of a life well spent, however short. Rare qualities like contentment, self-acceptance, inner calm, and compassion can be developed over time. Such qualities are sometimes hard to find in those who appear to be "successful" and healthy. Hard times can really bring out the best in us if we are willing to use them to train our mind and transform our outlook. So we can see that illness is not necessarily a negative force, in fact it can be just the opposite; simply by changing our mind we can transform illness or any adverse condition into a meaningful opportunity to develop our own inner qualities. We never know what life is going to "throw" at us, but we can be ready for it if we are willing to be flexible, positive, and willing to accept difficulties and use them to become more whole and "healthy" human beings.

What is good health?

Good health is simply a state of mind. Some people have developed the capacity to be deeply happy and content in the most adverse situations, dealing with great physical or environmental difficulties and becoming stronger, more whole, and complete human beings because of it. Such people often become spiritually and mentally "healthy," perhaps more healthy, in the truest sense of the word, than Olympic athletes! Certainly our inner achievements are ultimately of more value than our external triumphs. Although their value is not as immediately obvious they are a real treasure and if we build on them and strive to develop our inner qualities we will find great peace and contentment in this life and far into the future.

Although material wealth and good health give us a sense of security this will be short lived. Sooner or later these things will be taken from us and certainly at the end of our life we will have to leave them behind. There is no reason why we should not enjoy these short-term pleasures but if we expect them to afford some lasting comfort and protection we will be disappointed. So we have to look elsewhere for some lasting happiness and security and the best place to start is within. What we gain from within, what we learn about ourselves, what good qualities we develop as we go through life will always be with us. If we are happy within, our outlook will be positive whatever our circumstances. If we can share this point of view with patients, clients, friends, family, or anyone we meet, either directly or through good example we are really giving them something of great value. To give this kind of wisdom is the wisest kindness.

Giving yourself regular time and space to look at your life and the way you are living it is really important. Regular meditation, prayer, walks in the country, whatever helps you to get in touch with yourself and develop a little wisdom and clarity is priceless. It helps you to see where you are going and what might be coming to meet you from the future. It is not as difficult to see into the future as you think. It is simply a task of knowing that if you do not change your way of living and being then the past will tend to repeat itself and the future is generally a simple projection of the present. If your life is gray and dull now, it will probably be gray and dull or worse in the future, especially if you do not make an effort to paint a little color into things. We cannot buy these inner qualities, yet they are of the highest value. No one can give them to you and fortunately no one can take them away. We have to make an effort to develop them and keep them. This can be achieved most easily if you are walking a spiritual path or a path to personal growth that is authentic, complete, tried, and tested. If you try to succeed alone or if you choose a path that is not genuine you may progress intermittently but eventually you may find you slip back in to your old patterns of negativity and self-doubt. Having someone special to guide you and support your progress and others to compare notes and share the journey with is a great help and a guarantee of success.

Nowadays many people are discontent and possess great inner poverty, even rich and famous people! Yet it is not difficult to find happiness within when someone points you in the right direction! Developing inner happiness and contentment is a great treasure that we can all have in abundance simply by understanding and changing our inner nature. In fact all you really need is a happy mind. Understanding the true causes of happiness and suffering is right at the heart of Buddhist philosophy. If you are interested in knowing more about this it is best to read appropriate books or consult a fully qualified and realized teacher (see Appendices 1 and 2). Many of the healing techniques that Buddha taught and practiced are still used to this day, including the well-known practices of the Medicine Buddha, the embodiment of all the Buddha's healing qualities. You can receive the empowerment of Medicine Buddha from a qualified Buddhist teacher, which can help you to create a special connection with this healing Buddha. You can then receive teachings on a simple meditation practice in order to use the blessings of the Healing Buddha to heal yourselves and others. Consult Appendix 1 if you wish to know more about this from a qualified teacher.

All we need is a happy mind

Complementary therapies should help you change your mind, not the world around you; by changing your mind all things change. Your perception of yourself, your environment, and others changes completely when you change your mind or when your mind is changed. You will never find lasting happiness by trying to manufacture a perfect world for yourself. You can try to find the best job, the right partner, the nicest house, or the fastest car and for a short time you may find some happiness in these things but if you are honest you know in your heart that this happiness will come to an end. It is not real happiness and often serves to create more problems than it solves. In fact, the amount of pain and unhappiness you experience when you are separated from these things will at the very least be proportionate to the amount of "attachment" you have to them. There is a strong relationship between "need" and pain. The more you need someone or something to make you happy the more pain you will experience when you are eventually parted from them.

We also spend much time and effort manipulating our world to get what we want, when we want it, when all the happiness and peace of mind we could wish for is literally under our noses! You know that if you are deeply unhappy no amount of money, possessions, or relationships can help. So again this shows us that happiness depends upon the mind not on external factors. Understanding this simple wisdom and taking it to heart should give you great hope because this realization is the root of great happiness and the essence of a true spiritual path. Learning to open your heart and mind and develop some simple wisdom and contentment is time well spent and the rewards for accumulating these inner treasures are fathomless. This is not some difficult or mystical task; it is very simple and natural and you can use complementary therapies to help you begin and complete this journey toward self-understanding and lasting peace of mind.

The real spiritual practitioner seeks self-understanding and lasting inner peace, the real meaning of good health. They realize that they have exactly the right conditions at present to start developing higher qualities within themselves. Whether you are rich or poor does not matter, what matters is that you make an effort to change from within. Simply by making a daily determination to be a little more tolerant, patient, kind, and helpful is a great step forward. Then if you can carry forward these determinations into your daily activities and remind yourself of your good intentions especially when you are challenged by your own impatience or selfishness then you will begin to make real progress. You may wonder what relevance all this has to reflexology. Well, if you want to be a good healer or therapist you need to understand what good health is, then you will know how to help people achieve it. For the external practice of reflexology to be truly effective it should be combined with the healer's inner qualities and knowledge of the human condition. Just being in the presence of a healer with a little wisdom and compassion is really of more benefit than a thousand treatments from someone with a poor motivation.

Good motivation

If your motives are good, even if you make mistakes, the results will be beneficial right from your very first treatment. It also useful to remember that there is a right and a wrong time for giving advice. When people are not ready to change their minds and move toward good health then bombarding them with well-intentioned advice can be a real turn-off; we all know this! So wisdom dictates that a gentle approach, patience, and a good listening ear need to be employed until a patient naturally seeks knowledge for a new perspective on an old problem. A wise farmer will not throw good seed on poor ground; when the ground is fertile it is the right time to plant! You also have to be careful that a sense of wisdom does not breed arrogance or some subtle sense of superiority. Some eastern philosophies teach that the best healers are those who always regard the welfare of others, especially their patients, as most important. This sense of humility, that many of the great spiritual teachers like Jesus and Buddha displayed, is a very rare and great quality. It really allows you to get close to others and helps them to feel comfortable with you. A sense of superiority is a real barrier to the development of any healing relationship.

The nature of karma

The law of karma explains that the root causes of all our major and minor problems are our own previous negative actions of body, speech, and mind returning to us as illness, poverty, ignorance, or any other type of unpleasant experience. The word karma directly translates as "action" or what we intentionally create mentally, verbally, and/or physically. The laws of karma teach that whatever we create or give out comes back to us sooner or later, just like a boomerang! These negative actions may have been performed many lifetimes ago and it is only now that we may be experiencing the effects or repercussions. We might think that we could never have committed serious negative actions like harming others but in each of our previous lives we were almost completely different to the kind of person we are now. If we met ourselves from a previous life we would not recognize ourselves at all, it would be like meeting a complete stranger.

Deep within our very subtle mind we carry the memories, tendencies, and imprints of all our previous lives. When the conditions are right our previous actions of body, speech, and mind will return to us as positive or negative experiences, depending on whether they were well intentioned and beneficial or otherwise. From a Buddhist perspective, to fully heal and prevent future illness we must remove the root causes or the seeds of past negative actions from deep within the mind, before they ripen as unpleasant experiences. We could just as easily say that any person is simply the results of his previous actions ripening as pleasant or unpleasant characteristics and experiences. However, because one person is experiencing happiness and good fortune does not necessarily mean they are superior to others or that they have been kinder or more giving in previous lives. We all have an infinite amount of accumulated karma because we have had countless previous lives. We have all been good and bad people in previous lives so we don't know what karma will ripen next; it might be pleasant, it might not.

There is no grand plan or great scheme; life is simply a "karmic lottery." If the conditions are right any sort of karma could ripen, anything could happen to us if we have created the causes – we do not know what is round the corner. We know this is a fact of life – bad things can happen to good people and vice versa. A murderer can be reborn as a king in his next life if he has the karma from a previous life for that to happen. He may experience many fortunate rebirths in wealthy and loving families until eventually the karma of murdering catches up with him. Fortunately we can protect ourselves from our own karma by completely purifying it before it ripens. We cannot escape the law of karma simply by not believing it – it is a fact of life.

Healing through acceptance

Experience tells that we cannot always expect things to go our way. Sometimes no matter how hard we try we cannot escape or remove the effects of heavy negative karma that might be ripening in the form of a serious, possibly life-threatening, illness. This is a fact of life that can be difficult to accept. Of course, we can use reflexology and other therapies to help us deal with such challenging situations but we also have to be realistic and mature. Sometimes we simply have to accept what is happening to us and stop fighting. Developing a peaceful and happy mind is possible even in the face of great hardship. Learning to accept the things we cannot change and developing compassion for others who may be feeling for us shows great wisdom and maturity. Accepting difficulties with a peaceful and patient mind actually causes negative karma to be purified and exhausted much more quickly than if we develop anger, frustration, or sadness. Of course we may go through these emotions initially on the path to acceptance but if we "stay there" too long we are only making a difficult situation worse for ourselves and for those we love.

Any illness, before manifesting on the physical or conscious level, initially arises from the very subtle or deepest levels of mind, which are presently sub-conscious to most people. Ultimately we can only remove the true causes of illness by knowing, experiencing, and purifying our very subtle mind of all the potential seeds of illness planted or created by our own past negative actions in previous lives. This is our karma. However, even when these seeds have ripened or been removed the mental imprints of these past actions still remain in the mind, like footprints in the sand, and these create the mental tendencies to walk the same path again or commit similar negative actions in the future. These imprints must also be removed if we want to fully prevent illness or other negative experiences coming our way in this and future lives. We can do this by completely purifying our very subtle mind and developing a special type of wisdom, understanding the true nature of reality or in other words gaining "enlightenment." This is not some far-off, unattainable spiritual goal, the potential for us to achieve this is in our very nature – we just need someone to point us in the right direction! One tried and tested way toward enlightenment is through practicing the simple and clear meditation techniques that Buddha taught. You do not have to become Buddhist to learn these – they are open and available to anyone and they are ideally suited to your needs whatever your circumstances and commitments. In fact you do not need to change your lifestyle at all, only your mind! (See Appendix 1.)

The source of all suffering

So the main cause of illness is negative karma ripening when the correct conditions are in place. But what causes us to create negative karma? The simple answer to this is that "our selfish mind causes us to create negative karma." Likewise a *selfless* mind causes us to create positive karma, which will come back to us as a pleasant experience in the future and then we will also find it easier to repeat this tendency to be kind, thoughtful, and selfless again and again, bringing greater and greater good fortune and happiness.

Thinking of the welfare of others is a great source of future happiness and thinking of our own welfare is a source of future suffering. Even in the short term transferring our attention toward others and working for their benefit can take our mind off our own problems and cause us to be less introverted and self-obsessed. The more we worry about a problem the bigger it gets but the more we concern ourselves with helping others the less energy and time we give to our own worries and the weaker and less demanding they become. All the great spiritual teachers have taught and encouraged this; they knew that the source of all happiness is caring for others, all others, equally.

If we understand and accept the laws of karma we can gain great personal satisfaction from knowing that selfless actions not only benefit others but will also cause us to experience good fortune in the future. The main factor in creating karma is our true intention or motivation. Many people might appear to be altruistic on the outside, always doing good turns for others, but if their motivation is selfish, perhaps because they want others to like them, then this will not create a good karmic "return" in the future. Conversely, leading a very normal life with a pure motivation will lead to great future happiness.

What causes us to perform selfish actions? What causes us to think and act in a selfish way? If we can understand the answer to this then we are truly on the way to solving all our problems and finding a lasting cure to any present or potential future illness. We act instinctively and naturally to benefit ourselves because we think we are more important than others. Our sense of "self" is very dear to us and we cherish it deeply and in many subtle ways. We do not realize how deeply we cherish ourselves until we are faced with situations that frighten or challenge our sense of "self." So we have a strong sense of self, a strong sense that we truly exist and that this "self" is the most important thing in the universe. The fact that we grasp at this sense of "self," ego, or "I" and believe it to truly exist is the source of all our present and future problems. If we could realize our true nature and abandon the inner ignorance or lack of inner clarity or wisdom that gives rise to the sense of a very important "self" we could solve all our problems and experience complete and lasting happiness and freedom from suffering forever. This may sound unrealistic, unattainable, or even bizarre! But this message usually strikes a chord even in the most cynical heart.

Our mind can be compared to a glass of sparkling water, the constant stream of bubbles floating to the surface are like our thoughts and feelings. It appears that we "are" these thoughts and emotions that arise from within, as if they make up our identity and character or as if they are the "real me." Our true nature is more like the water itself than the bubbles that arise in it; our essence or source in reality is closer to the space between our thoughts and feelings. Ultimately this inner realization, understanding our own true nature, can become the universal cure for all illness and suffering.

How can we free ourselves and others from the effects of illness and the potential for future illness and all forms of suffering? The old biblical saying of "Physician heal thyself" is very relevant here. We cannot truly help others until we have healed ourselves and a true healing is one that is complete and lasting and comes from within. We can only accomplish this by realizing our true nature and becoming all that we can be; then we will have the wisdom and power to help others achieve the same state of complete happiness and permanent freedom from any kind of problem or unhappiness. Sounds boring? But then is any kind of suffering really exciting or interesting? To reach this special destination we have to find a path that leads there clearly and directly. Buddha taught such a path thousands of years ago; many people realized his teachings then and found great happiness and inner peace as a result. Because we have an unbroken and pure lineage of these teachings and instructions many people from all backgrounds and religions today are also finding this timeless wisdom invaluable and completely relevant to the problems they face. Ultimately Buddhism is really "Truism" – it simply tells us the way things are, the way things will be, and the way we can improve them! If you ever wanted to know who you are, why you're here, and where you're going simply pick up a good book on Buddhism! It will be a map of reality! (See Appendix 2.) Having said that, Buddhism does not have a monopoly on the truth, and many of Buddha's teachings are reflected in all of the great world religions and spiritual paths to truth and happiness. We cannot say that one is superior or better than another – they all have good qualities and perhaps we can say that they are all leading in a similar direction and come from the same "nameless" source. As individuals we have to find one that we feel comfortable with and one that we feel shines with clarity and truth.

The power of compassion

The quality of your mind can have a very definitive effect on your ability to heal others. The mind is quite a subtle object and the effects of the thoughts and intentions that accompany your actions are not easily revealed unless you are familiar with your inner world. However, you can prove this in another way. If someone were to practice reflexology and they were in a very negative frame of mind, perhaps impatient or distracted and not that bothered about the welfare of the person they were treating, then this would obviously have a profound effect on the treatment. The client would sense this and not be at ease and leave with little faith in the treatment. So you can see that many "doors" are already closing and the chance of a successful treatment is reduced. Conversely if the therapist has his or her client's best interests at heart and has a mind of great compassion then this will naturally lead to a successful treatment and also give the client confidence in the therapist and therefore the treatment.

We also have to look again at karma to gain some clarity on this issue. Obviously the karma of the client and therapist is the key factor in the possibility of a successful treatment. There are two conditions that they can establish that will help the karma of a successful treatment to ripen. From the therapist's side the mind of pure compassion is vital and from the patient's side the minds of patience, faith in the therapist, therapy, or the healing "energy," and the wish to be well are also vital. Even if you only have a little of these qualities then that will give reflexology enough "room" to work well! If the patient themselves can try to develop more compassion for others this will also aid their own healing process. We may wonder why this is so. Well, the opposite of compassion is a selfish mind and selfish minds are one of the conditions that can encourage the karma of illness to ripen. Conversely, a wish to use your life well and to help others whenever possible will help the karma of good health to ripen. It is important to stress that this is not a guarantee of good health – many compassionate people suffer from illness, it is simply another "condition" that can influence health.

Good or bad karma can only ripen if we have created the causes by planting the seeds of this karma by our actions of body, speech, and mind in previous lives. This is why some very negative people never get ill and have long lives and why some very positive people get ill and sometimes die young. It is all about causes and conditions: if we have not created the causes to be ill or we have removed them through inner purification, whatever conditions we create we will not become ill. There is one more advantage in trying to develop our compassion and that is if selfish actions lead to future suffering then compassion must lead to great health and happiness in the future.

Healing conditions

Regular reflexology can greatly enhance your health and protect you from future illness by preventing the potential causes of illness arising from deep within the mind and creating the necessary conditions for good health to return. Illness can only arise from within the mind if the right "conditions" are present. Likewise, a potential illness can be prevented from arising by eliminating stress, poor diet, depressing environments, and most importantly negative states of mind and poor quality internal energies. Using reflexology can be a protection against negative minds and impure internal energy, the major conditions that cause illness to arise. So reflexology can work in two ways: to heal existing problems and prevent future ones arising. This understanding coupled with a positive and compassionate nature can create a very special healing potential.

10

Hand reflexology with essential oils

This chapter gives an insight into the history and practice of aromatherapy, a special healing therapy that combines wonderfully with hand and foot reflexology. The following information is provided by www.aworldofaromatherapy.com. There are some excellent ideas here for the different ways to use aromatherapy oils in between full treatments. When you use aromatherapy oils during a full treatment you can either use them throughout the treatment, or just at the start during the warm-up if you do not want to put too much healing pressure on the body. As mentioned, the healing process cannot be rushed, especially with serious illness, so a gentle approach is recommended. Combining two powerful healing techniques like reflexology and aromatherapy needs to be done carefully. You can also give the patient or client a bottle containing the same aromatherapy oils to take home with them. Perhaps they know someone who could give them a neck, shoulder, and back massage with it or you could teach them some simple hand reflexology techniques to practice at home. They could also put a few drops in their bath or use a diffuser to fill the air with the fragrance. For a complete list of the most commonly used essential oils and what conditions they can be used for see Appendix 3.

In the beginning

With origins dating back 5000 years, aromatherapy is truly one of the oldest methods of holistic healing. Ancient man was dependent on his surroundings for everything from food to shelter and clothing. Being so keenly aware of everything around him, and how it could be used for survival, he quickly discovered methods to preserve food and treat ailments through herbs and aromatics. Aromatherapy, as it is practiced today, began with the Egyptians, who used the method of infusion to extract the oils from aromatic plants, which were used for medicinal and cosmetic purposes as well as embalming. At a similar time, ancient Chinese civilizations were also using some form of aromatics. Shen Nung's herbal book (dating back to approximately 2700 BC) contains detailed information on over 300 plants and their uses. Similarly, the Chinese used aromatics in religious ceremonies, by burning woods and incense to show respect to their Gods – a tradition that is still practiced today. The use of aromatics in China was linked to other ancient therapies, such as massage and acupressure.

Aromatherapy has also been used for many centuries in India. Ayurveda, the traditional medical system of India, uses dried and fresh herbs, as well as aromatic massage, as important aspects of treatment. The Greeks acquired most of their medical knowledge from the Egyptians and used it to further their own discoveries. They found that the fragrance of some flowers was stimulating while others had relaxing properties. The use of olive oil as the base oil absorbed the aroma from the herbs or flowers and the perfumed oil was then used for both cosmetic and medicinal purposes.

The Romans learned from the Greeks and became well known for scented baths followed by massage with aromatic oils. The popularity of aromatics led to the establishment of trade routes, which allowed the Romans to import "exotic" oils and spices from distant lands such as India and Arabia. With the decline of the Roman Empire, the use of aromatics faded and the knowledge of their use was virtually lost in Europe during the Dark Ages.

Rediscovery of a healing art

One of the few places where the tradition of aromatherapy continued was in monasteries, where monks used plants from herbal gardens to produce infused oils, herbal teas, and medicines. At the time of the plague, and during the Middle Ages, it was discovered that certain aromatic derivatives helped to prevent the spread of infection, and others, such as cedar and pine, were burnt to fumigate homes and streets. The revival of the use of essential oils is credited to a Persian physician and philosopher known as Avicenna, who lived from AD 980 to AD 1037. The Arabs initiated a method of extraction known as distillation, and study of the therapeutic use of plants once again became popular in the universities. The knowledge of distillation spread to their invading forces during the Crusades, and the lost process was once again returned to Europe. By AD 1200, essential oils were being produced in Germany and were based mainly on herbs and spices brought from Africa and the Far East. When South America was invaded by the conquistadors even more medicinal plants and aromatic oils were discovered, and the wide variety of medicinal plants found in Montezuma's gardens provided a basis for many new and important remedies and treatments. Throughout the northern continent, Native Americans were using aromatic oils and producing their own herbal remedies, which were discovered when settlers began to make their way across the plains of the New World. Although herbs and aromatics had been used in other world cultures for many centuries, it was not until the nineteenth century that scientists in Europe and Great Britain began researching the effects of essential oils on humans. It was the French chemist, Rene Maurice Gattefosse, who discovered the healing powers of lavender oil after burning his hand in his laboratory. He published a book on the anti-microbial effects of the oils in 1937 and the term "Aromatherapy" was born. Essential oils are the highly concentrated essences of aromatic plants. Aromatherapy is the art of using these oils to promote healing of the body and the mind.

The basics of aromatherapy

Each of the essential oils used in aromatherapy can be used either alone or in combinations to create a desired effect. Before using essential oils as part of an aromatherapy treatment, it is important to understand the effect that the oils have, and how they work. The oils are found in different parts of the plant, such as the flowers, twigs, leaves, and bark, or in the rind of fruit. For example, in roses it is found in the flowers, in basil it is in the leaves, in sandalwood in the wood, and so on. The methods used to extract the oil are time consuming and expensive and require a high degree of expertise. Given that it takes in excess of 220 pounds of rose petals to produce only 4 or 5 teaspoonfuls of oil, it is a process probably best left to professionals! Due to the large quantity of plant material required, pure essential oils are expensive, but they are also highly effective – only a few drops at a time are required to achieve the desired effect. Synthetic oils are available at a lesser price, but they simply do not have the healing power of the natural oils.

How essential oils work

Essential oils have an immediate impact on our sense of smell, also known as "olfaction." When essential oils are inhaled, olfactory receptor cells are stimulated and the impulse is transmitted to the emotional center of the brain, or "limbic system."

The limbic system is connected to areas of the brain linked to memory, breathing, and blood circulation, as well as the endocrine glands, which regulate hormone levels in the body. The properties of the oil, the fragrance and its effects, determine stimulation of these systems. When used in massage, essential oils are not only inhaled, but absorbed through the skin as well. They penetrate the tissues and find their way into the bloodstream where they are transported to the organs and systems of the body.

Essential oils have differing rates of absorption, generally between 20 minutes and two hours, so to ensure maximum effectiveness it is probably best not to bathe or shower directly following a massage.

The notes of essential oils

Essential oils are often described by their "note." The three categories of classification are top note, middle note, and base note, and these terms relate to the rate at which they evaporate – or how long the fragrance will last.

Top notes are the most stimulating and uplifting oils. They are strongly scented, but the perfume lasts only for approximately 3-24 hours. Examples of top note oils are basil, bergamot, clary sage, coriander, eucalyptus, lemongrass, neroli, peppermint, sage, and thyme.

Middle notes are the next longest lasting, at about 2-3 days, and affect the metabolic and body functions. The perfume is less potent than that of top note oils.

Examples of middle note oils are balm, chamomile, fennel, geranium, hyssop, juniper, lavender, and rosemary.

Base notes are the slowest oils to evaporate, lasting up to one week. They have a sweet, soothing scent and a relaxing, comforting effect on the body. Examples of Base note oils are cedarwood, clove, frankincense, ginger, jasmine, rose, and sandalwood.

Creating aromatherapy blends

To create a balanced perfume, a combination of all three notes will produce the best results. It is important to state that when making aromatherapy blends, there are no fixed rules. The more familiar you become with the fragrances and their effects, the easier it will be to create combinations that are right for you!

The use of essential oils in massage is a fantastic way to

maximize the healing power of the massage itself. When combined with essential oils, a massage can have a powerful calming or energizing effect, depending on the oil chosen and the strokes of the masseur (quick movements will stimulate and slow movements relax).

When using essential oils in massage, always dilute the oils in a carrier oil prior to application to the skin. As we've said before, essential oils are very powerful concentrates, and unless indicated otherwise, should not be directly applied to the skin or irritation can result.

Carrier oils

Carrier oils are just that. They are the oils that carry the essential oil. There is a wide variety available including the following:

- **Almond Oil** – very easily absorbed by the skin, very smooth, has little smell, keeps well, contains vitamin D, and has beneficial effects on hair, dry skin, and brittle nails
- **Apricot kernel Oil** – light, contains Vitamin A, particularly good for use on the face if the skin is dry or aging
- **Avocado Oil** – heavy, rich in nutrients, very good for dry, aging, and sensitive skins
- **Evening Primrose Oil** – helpful for skin conditions such as eczema and psoriasis, only keeps for about two months after opening
- **Grapeseed Oil** – light, good for oily skin, one of the least expensive oils
- **Hazelnut Oil** – penetrates the skin very easily and is deeply nourishing
- **Jojoba Oil** – light, rich in vitamin E, beneficial for spots, acne, dandruff, and dry scalp
- **Olive Oil** – can be used in a pinch, but has a strong smell

which may compete with the essential oil
- **Peach Kernel Oil** – light, contains vitamins A and E, very good for the face
- **Soya Oil** – easily absorbed, rich in vitamin E
- **Sunflower Oil** – contains essential fatty acids, rich in vitamin E, has a slightly nutty smell
- **Wheatgerm Oil** – contains vitamins A, B, C, and E, firms and tones the skin, reduces blemishes, can help to reduce scar tissue and stretch marks, has a strong smell

The massage

When combining oils to be used in massage, have the proper supplies on hand. Dark bottles (brown, blue, etc.) in a 2oz size work very well, and can be obtained with relative ease. Using a small funnel, fill the container half full until you have about 1oz of carrier oil. To the carrier oil, add 12-15 drops of essential oil and place the lid on the container. Shake well (the container – not you!!). You can use only one essential oil or combine up to three of your choice to comprise the 12-15 drops. And there you have it! Your very own blend of massage oil!

Tip: Make small quantities as outlined above or you may end up with leftovers – blended oils will turn rancid fairly quickly. Store in a cool dark place with the lid tightly closed and they will last up to three months. Let your nose be your guide – if the blend no longer smells good, consider a fresh mix!

In the air

There are a variety of ways to fill your surroundings with the pleasant aromas of essential oils. They can be added to humidifiers, vaporizers, the molten wax of a candle, the dish of a diffuser (mixed with water), or even combined with water in a spray bottle. Simply add a few drops of your favorite oil, or see our recipes below for some helpful suggestions:

Recipe for a fresh, clean smell in the air: 1 drop cedarwood, 3 drops pine, 2 drops rosemary.

Recipe to induce sleep: 2 drops chamomile, 2 drops lavender, 2 drops neroli.

Steam inhalation (not recommended for asthmatics): place a few drops of essential oil into a bowl of very hot water. Lean over the bowl (approximately eight inches from the water, or choose a comfortable distance for you), and drape a towel over your head. Inhale the steam deeply for 5-10 minutes (again, the length of time should be determined by your comfort level), remove the towel from your head, and blot the moisture from your face.

Once you are finished, leaving the bowl and its contents out in the open will continue to release the healing steam and aromas into the air, so don't be so quick to dump it down the sink!

Recipe for cold and flu using steam inhalation: 3 drops eucalyptus.

In the bath

Run a warm bath and ensure the door and windows are closed. When the tub is sufficiently filled, add up to 10 drops of essential oil to the water, circulating it throughout. As the oil is moved, the scent will rise with the steam of the water. Now get in, take your time, and enjoy the wonderful aroma while you soak!

Recipe for a relaxing and calming bath: 2 drops bergamot, 2 drops cedarwood.

Recipe to relieve nervousness: 6 drops geranium, 4 drops basil.

Recipe for insomnia: 3 drops chamomile, 2 drops lavender, 2 drops neroli, 2 drops marjoram.

Recipe for an energizing bath: 3 drops rosemary, 2 drops lemon, 2 drops frankincense.

For tired, sore, worn out feet, the aromatherapy foot bath provides great relief! Fill a container (big enough to house both of your feet) with very warm water and add a few drops of essential oil. Sit back, relax, and give those barking dogs a rest!

Recipe for aching feet: 3 drops peppermint.

As mentioned above, a full list of the most commonly used essential oils is given in Appendix 3. By using this list and the above guidelines you should be able to identify or formulate a particular essential oil or combination of oils that will suit your own or your patient's or client's requirements.

11

Meditations for health and well-being

If we develop a little experience of the benefits of meditation we can share this with others by teaching clients, patients, friends, or family how to relax the body and mind and generate a positive outlook. The beauty of teaching a patient a simple relaxation technique is that if they can do this a little every day in between reflexology treatments this will greatly assist their mental, emotional, and physical healing. The benefits of regular meditation are now well known. We gain improved health and well-being in many ways, levels of stress are greatly reduced, and positive, peaceful, and confident states of mind are easily generated. There are many scientific studies to validate the healing power of meditation alone. With regular meditation, among other benefits, many people report increased mental clarity, more energy, reduced levels of stress, and a feeling of inner peace. So it can be as good for the therapist as for the patient! Meditation is a very simple, natural, and powerful way of realizing our abilities to become more whole, healthy, and happy human beings from within. To gain the most from meditation we really need to find a local meditation group that is led by an experienced teacher from an authentic tradition. (See Appendix 1.) However, this chapter is designed to give the reader an introduction to meditation and if you follow the instructions carefully you can gain great benefit from practicing for just 10 to 15 minutes per day.

Breathing meditation

You need at least 10 minutes to do this kind of meditation; early morning is often best when you are fresh as this can really help you start and continue the day in a positive way. The room you use should be peaceful and clean and if you have a particular religious belief you can set up a small shrine or altar with holy pictures, Scriptures, and offerings. This serves as a spiritual focal point and helps to build and hold a good quality of energy or atmosphere in your meditation space. If you intentionally honor, clean, and look after this space regularly and treat it with respect, you are definitely creating the causes for your meditations to gradually become clearer and deeper, with long-lasting benefits. Your meditation posture is very important: you can meditate sitting up in a chair with your back straight, but not tense, your feet flat on the floor, and hands resting in your lap, or you can sit on a floor cushion in a traditional meditation posture.

To begin, relax the body by slowly mentally "scanning" for tension and releasing it. Begin at the top of the head and slowly work down through the various muscle groups and parts of the body until you reach the toes. Then bring your attention to your breathing and particularly to the sensation at the tip of the nostrils, becoming aware of the cool air coming in and the warm air going out. Focus your mind on this gentle sensation completely. The gentle sensation of the breath in the nostrils is your "object" of meditation – try to keep your mind gently but firmly focused on this one thing. As soon as you notice that you have lost the object of meditation – you might be distracted by sounds or thoughts – find it again and try to hold it for as long as possible. This type of meditation focuses the mind and improves your clarity and concentration. In fact this simple breathing meditation, if practiced for 10 or 15 minutes daily, can greatly improve your quality of life by giving a clear and peaceful mind. Every time you "lose" your object of meditation and begin thinking about other things, simply bring your attention back to the sensations of breathing. If you have no experience of meditation it can be helpful to practice just the breathing meditation for several days or weeks before trying anything else. The breathing meditation is the foundation for all further meditation so it is important to persevere with a patient and realistic approach, not expecting amazing results overnight, but just training gradually over weeks and months and years.

Meditation on compassion

This kind of meditation has two main aspects: "contemplation" is the process you use to "find" your object of meditation, in this case a feeling of compassion, and "placement" is the act of "holding" or concentrating on this feeling.

To develop compassion you can first contemplate how the opposite of compassion – anger or hatred – causes so many problems in the world: the selfish mind of anger is responsible for all conflicts and wars; if no one ever experienced anger we would live in a very peaceful world. Contemplate how angry or selfish thoughts and feelings have caused us and others many problems and great unhappiness in the past and consider how wonderful it would be to be free from these heavy negative minds. Then when you naturally feel a strong wish to release these feelings and develop the opposing positive quality of love, try to "hold" and encourage these positive intentions. Then contemplate the problems that others experience in their lives. You can think about people you know who are very unhappy or about situations you have heard about or seen on TV where people or animals are suffering. When a feeling of compassion arises in the mind toward these beings hold on to it for as long as possible and try to mix your mind with it completely, almost as if you have become compassion.

Toward the end of the meditation make a firm determination to act to help others whenever you can. This determination is the final goal of your meditation and you should try to make it as deep and heartfelt as possible and try to remember that determination throughout the rest of the day. The key to successful meditation is to consistently make a strong inner determination to let go of negative and damaging ways of living and being and develop more positive, harmonious, and constructive ones. If your mind wanders during meditation simply return to the contemplation until you find the object of meditation again, then hold it for as long as possible. You are actually training or encouraging yourself to eventually think and feel this way quite naturally. When you "hold" an object of meditation you should not strain the mind – it should feel natural, as if your mind has completely mixed or become "one" with the object of meditation, i.e. your wish to be more tolerant, patient, or compassionate. By regularly developing these deep wishes to change for the better you will definitely become more positive, happy, content, and considerate. Throughout the day, whenever you become aware that negative feelings or thoughts, like worry or impatience, are about to arise in the mind you can prevent them having influencing by recalling your earlier good intentions. In this way you can train in meditation all the time, not just while you are sitting on your cushion and your wisdom and happiness will gradually increase and your daily problems will steadily decrease. This ancient tried and tested way of dealing with life's problems, if practiced correctly and regularly, is a guaranteed solution and unlike other modern methods of finding happiness, addiction to it produces very healthy results!

Learning and sharing your experiences with others, meditating in a group and having the opportunity to ask questions, can add greatly to your enjoyment and progress. Also, having a teacher who is a living example of what you can achieve through meditation is a constant inspiration and encouragement to your own developing practice. If you want to find a meditation group in your area see Appendix 1. If you do a little meditation every day good results will accumulate, you will become more relaxed and more able to enjoy life fully; gradually you will become a true source of wisdom, compassion, and inner strength.

OM AH HUM meditation

Although this mantra is very short it is one of the most blessed mantras, representing or expressing of the body, speech, and mind of all the Buddhas. It is very helpful if you can remember this while you are doing the meditation and especially develop the wish to transform your own body, speech, and mind into that of an enlightened being for the benefit of others. Developing this motivation before you begin to meditate is very important, it will make your meditation more powerful and you create the karma to become an enlightened being in the future. Intention is everything. If you live your live with the intention of finding happiness for yourself this is quite a narrow mind, considering how many living beings there are, who all wish to be happy. If you can learn to focus on the welfare of others more than your own this shows great wisdom, as this is the mind that will in fact bring you most happiness, but most importantly it will bring more peace to the world and have a very positive influence on others.

In this meditation you combine breathing meditation and mantra recitation. As with all meditation, you need a peaceful environment and to sit comfortably with your back fairly straight but not too straight and your hands resting gently in your lap. Breathe naturally through the nostrils and spend some time mentally checking through the body from head to foot to see if you can find any tension. Allow yourself to fully relax and simply imagine any tension draining away down through the body and into the floor. When you are fully relaxed bring your attention to your breathing, becoming aware of the natural rise and fall of the breath.

To develop some clarity in the mind for a few minutes you

can focus on the gentle sensation at the tip of the nostrils as the cool air comes in and the warm air goes out. When your mind is relaxed and focused you can begin to mentally recite the OM AH HUM mantra. As you inhale mentally recite OM, then hold your breath at your heart for a short time and mentally recite AH, them exhale and mentally recite HUM while breathing out. Repeat this process for as long as you wish. This very simple meditation brings profound results. If you practice for 10 to 15 minutes every day, in time your mind will become more and more peaceful and less distracted. In time you may even find it difficult to become agitated or unhappy! Inner peace will become your natural state of mind.

12

Final thoughts

I would like to mention three other therapies that work well with hand and foot reflexology. These are Reiki, the Metamorphic Technique, and Bach Flower Remedies (see Appendices 4, 5, and 6 for more details). These are complete and unique therapies in their own right but are especially relevant to reflexologists. They combine with reflexology in a wonderful way, as does aromatherapy. They are very easy to learn and yet very powerful and profound healing techniques. If you are interested in becoming a dedicated healer I would definitely recommend spending a year learning hand and foot reflexology at a recognized college and then back this up with learning Reiki and Metamorphic Technique. The basics of these therapies can be learned in only one or two days. If you do this and combine your practice with a basic knowledge of aromatherapy and Bach Flower Therapy through your own study, you will be in an excellent position to benefit many, many people.

Not many people practice reflexology for the money! If you want to dedicate your life to the accumulation of material wealth then reflexology is probably not the path for you. However, if you are interested in using your time to help cure, relieve, and prevent illness and you want to practice a therapy that is powerful, gentle, and intimate yet non-invasive then reflexology might be your vocation. You will certainly gain great personal satisfaction from seeing the pleasure and peace others derive from your healing actions, paid or unpaid. Basically if you have a genuine concern for the welfare of others you will be a good healer.

Appendix 1
Meditation

The demand for a lasting solution to the problems of stress and anxiety, created by the nature of today's "material" society, has led to the setting up of meditation groups in almost every town and city. These groups vary in content and in their spiritual origin, so it is important to find one that you feel comfortable with, one that is run by a fully qualified teacher, and one that teaches a recognized and correct "path" true to the origins of meditation.

Buddhist meditation

Most meditation groups can trace their origins back to Buddha, who lived over 2000 years ago. He was born into one of the richest and most powerful royal families in India and spent the first 29 years of his life living as a prince. However, despite having all the health, wealth, and good relationships he could wish for he still felt incomplete and he could also see a great need in others for a real solution to life's problems. Finally he came to understand that most people look for happiness in the wrong place! He felt sure that true, lasting happiness could be found simply by understanding and developing the mind. He decided to give up his inheritance and devote the rest of his life to attaining the ultimate state of wisdom and happiness, so that he could share this with others. All Buddha's teachings were recorded and passed down and to this day we have a pure, unbroken lineage of the path to full enlightenment. This lineage is now firmly established in the West. We do not have to travel far to find it!

New Kadampa Tradition

One of the largest international Buddhist organizations is the New Kadampa Tradition. Established in 1976 by Tibetan meditation master, Geshe Kelsang Gyatso Rinpoche, its purpose is "to present the mainstream of Buddhist teachings in a way that is relevant and immediately applicable to the contemporary Western way of life." Most cities and towns in the UK have an NKT residential center or meditation group and many others are opening in the USA, Europe, and all over the world (see Appendix 2 for books by Geshe Kelsang Gyatso on Buddhism and Buddhist practice). To find your nearest Buddhist center, or if you would like a teacher to give an introductory talk on Buddhism in your area, please contact:

New Kadampa Tradition
The Kadampa Meditation Center,
Sweeney Road,
Glen Spey NY 12737, USA

Tel: (845) 856-9000
Toll free: 1-877-kadampa (1-877-523-2672)
Fax: (845) 856-2110
E-mail: info@kadampacenter.org
www.kadampa.net

In UK: NEW KADAMPA TRADITION
Conishead Priory,
Ulverston,
Cumbria,
LA12 9QQ,
Tel/Fax: 01229 588533 (within UK).
Email: kadampa@dircon.co.uk
www.kadampa.net

Appendix 2
Books on Buddhism

For beginners and more experienced practitioners, the following books are written by Geshe Kelsang Gyatso and published by Tharpa Publications:

Transform Your Life – A Blissful Journey
Introduction to Buddhism – An Explanation of the Buddhist Way of Life
The New Meditation Handbook – A Practical Guide to Meditation
Universal Compassion – Transforming Your Life Through Love and Compassion
Eight Steps to Happiness – Transform Your Mind, Transform Your Life
Joyful Path of Good Fortune – The Complete Buddhist Path to Enlightenment
Meaningful to Behold – The Bodhisattva's Way of Life
Guide to the Bodhisattva's Way of Life – A Buddhist Poem for Today

There are many other more advanced and in-depth titles on Buddhism available from Tharpa Publications; they also produce Buddhist art reproductions, tapes, talking books, and books in Braille. For more information visit www.tharpa.com.

Appendix 3

Commonly used essential oils

The following information is kindly provided by www. aworldofaromatherapy.com. Any of the oils can be obtained through the website or at your local natural health shop

BASIL
Effects: uplifting and stimulating
Aroma: top note
Scent: fresh, sweet, spicy
Combines well with: citrus oils, frankincense, geranium
Properties: analgesic, antidepressant, antiseptic, antispasmodic, uplifting
Uses: bronchitis, colds, constipation, insect bites, mental fatigue, migraine, nervous tension, rheumatism, sinus congestion
Contra-indications: May cause irritation to sensitive skin. Use well diluted. Not to be used during pregnancy.

BERGAMOT
Effects: refreshing and uplifting
Aroma: top note
Scent: sweet, spicy
Combines well with: chamomile, geranium, lavender
Properties: antidepressant, antiseptic, antispasmodic

Uses: abscesses, acne, boils, chicken pox, colds, cold sores,
     cystitis, flatulence, loss of appetite, mouth infections, sore
     throat
Contra-indications: Bergamot is a photosensitizer (increases the
     skins reaction to sunlight making it more likely to burn) so
     it should not be used when exposed to sunlight or tanning
     beds. Bergamot has antispasmodic properties and therefore
     should be avoided during pregnancy.

BLACK PEPPER
Effects: stimulating
Aroma: middle note
Scent: warm, peppery
Combines well with: lavender, rosemary, sandalwood
Properties: diuretic, expectorant, stimulant
Uses: chilblains, colds, constipation, digestive problems,
     flatulence, heartburn, indigestion, loss of appetite, muscle
     aches and pains, sinus congestion
Contra-indications: Black pepper may irritate sensitive skin.
     Use well diluted. Avoid use during pregnancy.

CAJEPUT
Effects: clearing
Aroma: top note
Scent: camphor, medicinal
Combines well with: eucalyptus, rosemary, tea tree
Properties: analgesic, antiseptic, expectorant, insecticide
Uses: bronchitis, colds, earache, laryngitis, lung congestion,
     neuralgia, rheumatism, skin conditions (such as acne),
     toothache
Contra-indications: In high concentrations, Cajeput may cause
     skin irritation.

CHAMOMILE
Effects: soothing, relaxing
Aroma: middle note

Scent: sweet, herbal, fruity

Combines well with: bergamot, geranium, Lavender

Properties: analgesic, antibacterial, antiseptic, digestive stimulant

Uses: acne, blisters, boils, colitis, depression, digestive problems, flatulence, gout, headaches, indigestion, irritable bowel syndrome, neuralgia, nervous tension (anxiety, fear), rheumatism, skin conditions (dermatitis, eczema, psoriasis)

Contra-indications: Chamomile may cause skin irritation. Not to be used in early pregnancy.

CEDARWOOD

Effects: soothing, strengthening

Aroma: base note

Scent: woody

Combines well with: bergamot, rosemary, sandalwood

Properties: anti-fungal, antiseptic, astringent, expectorant, sedative

Uses: arthritis, bronchitis, cellulite, cystitis, dandruff (blend with rosemary),

skin conditions (such as acne, eczema, oily skin)

Contra-indications: Cedarwood may cause skin irritation to sensitive skin. Do not use during pregnancy.

CLARY SAGE

Effects: warming

Aroma: top/middle note

Scent: sweet, spicy, herbal

Combines well with: geranium, lavender, rose

Properties: anti-inflammatory, antiseptic, antispasmodic, sedative

Uses: asthma, depression, digestive problems, exhaustion, muscle cramps and spasms, PMS relief, respiratory problems

Contra-indications: Do not use clary sage during pregnancy. Clary sage is highly sedative – do not use before driving or other activities requiring a high level of focus and concentration.

CLOVE
Effects: warming
Aroma: base/middle note
Scent: Sweet, spicy, fresh
Combines well with: lavender, orange, ylang ylang
Properties: analgesic, expectorant, stimulant
Uses: bronchitis, colds, indigestion, infected wounds, insect
    repellant, mouth sores, muscle and nerve tension, room
    disinfectant, toothache.
Contra-indications: Clove is highly irritating to the skin and
    must be diluted to concentrations less than 1% prior to use.

CYPRESS
Effects: relaxing, refreshing
Aroma: middle/base note
Scent: sweet, refreshing
Combines well with: citrus oils, juniper, lavender
Properties: antispasmodic, astringent, diuretic, expectorant
Uses: asthma, bronchitis, cough, edema, hemorrhoids,
    menopause symptoms,
menstrual symptoms, muscle and nerve tension, oily skin and/
    or hair
Rheumatism
Contra-indications: Cypress has antispasmodic properties and
    is therefore probably best avoided during pregnancy.

EUCALYPTUS
Effects: balancing, stimulating
Aroma: top/middle note
Scent: camphorous, woody
Combines well with: juniper, lavender, marjoram
Properties: analgesic, anti-inflammatory, antiseptic, antiviral,
    stimulant
Uses: air disinfectant, asthma, bronchitis, burns, cuts,
    decongestant, flu, headaches, insect repellant, muscle aches,
    rheumatism, sinusitis, skin ulcers, urinary infections, wounds

Contra-indications: Eucalyptus should not be used if you have high blood pressure or epilepsy and can be fatal if ingested.

FENNEL
Effects: clearing
Aroma: middle note
Scent: sweet, earthy
Combines well with: geranium, lavender, sandalwood
Properties: antiseptic, antispasmodic, diuretic, stimulant
Uses: digestive disorders, gout (combine with juniper), nervous tension
Contra-indications: Do not use fennel during pregnancy or if you have epilepsy. Fennel may irritate sensitive skin.

FRANKINCENSE
Effects: uplifting, relaxing
Aroma: base/middle note
Scent: sweet, warm
Combines well with: lavender, neroli, rose
Properties: analgesic, antidepressant, anti-inflammatory, antiseptic, expectorant
Uses: asthma, bronchitis, colds, healing wounds, tension, respiratory conditions, skin care (mature/aging skin), uterine tonic (can be used for heavy periods and massage following childbirth)
Contra-indications: None known.

GERANIUM
Effects: comforting, healing
Aroma: middle note
Scent: floral, sweet, earthy
Combines well with: chamomile, cypress, Juniper
Properties: anti-fungal, antiseptic, antispasmodic, diuretic
Uses: burns, eczema, edema, fluid retention, neuralgia, PMS symptoms (including swollen breasts), poor circulation, rheumatism, tonsillitis

Contra-indications: Geranium may irritate sensitive skin. Avoid use during pregnancy due to antispasmodic properties.

GINGER
Effects: warming
Aroma: top note
Scent: warm, spicy, woody
Combines well with: cedarwood, citrus oils, eucalyptus
Properties: analgesic, antidepressant, expectorant, stimulant
Uses: arthritis, bronchitis, catarrh, colds, colic, constipation, diarrhea, exhaustion, flatulence, flu, indigestion, poor circulation, rheumatism, sinusitis
Contra-indications: Ginger may irritate sensitive skin.

GRAPEFRUIT
Effects: refreshing
Aroma: top note
Scent: sweet, citrus
Combines well with: lavender, other citrus oils
Properties: antiseptic, astringent, diuretic, stimulant
Uses: anxiety, depression, digestive problems, water retention
Contra-indications: Grapefruit is a photosensitizer (increases the skin's reaction to sunlight making it more likely to burn) so it should not be used when exposed to sunlight or tanning beds.

HYSSOP
Effects: stimulating
Aroma: middle note
Scent: warm, sweet
Combines well with: fennel, lavender, tangerine
Properties: antiseptic, antispasmodic, astringent, diuretic, expectorant, stimulant
Uses: asthma, bronchitis, colds, cough, mental tension, sore throat, stomach cramps, water retention
Contra-indications: Hyssop should not be used during

pregnancy, or if you have high blood pressure or epilepsy.

JASMINE
Effects: soothing, relaxing
Aroma: base note
Scent: warm, floral
Combines well with: chamomile, citrus oils, rose
Properties: antidepressant, antiseptic, antispasmodic, expectorant
Uses: anxiety, catarrh, cough, headache, lack of confidence, laryngitis, mental tension, sensitive or dry skin
Contra-indications: Jasmine is generally agreeable with most, but some allergic reactions can occur. Jasmine should not be used during pregnancy because of its antispasmodic properties.

JUNIPER
Effects: cleansing, refreshing
Aroma: middle note
Scent: Fresh, woody, sweet
Combines well with: frankincense, lavender, rose
Properties: analgesic, astringent, diuretic, expectorant
Uses: acne, cellulite, cystitis, dermatitis, disinfectant, eczema (weeping), gout, muscle aches and pains, rheumatism, sores and ulcers
Contra-indications: Juniper should not be used during pregnancy or if you have severe kidney disease.

LAVENDER
Effects: calming, therapeutic
Aroma: middle note
Scent: floral, sweet, woody, herbal
Combines well with: clary sage, frankincense, geranium
Properties: analgesic, anti-inflammatory, antiseptic, diuretic, insecticide, sedative
Uses: acne, anxiety, bronchitis, burns, catarrh, chilblains,

circulatory problems, colds, dandruff, eczema, flu, headaches, insect bites, insomnia, muscle aches and pains, PMS symptoms, psoriasis, rheumatism, sinusitis, skin problems, sunburn, tension, throat infection, wounds and sores

Contra-indications: Lavender should not be used during the early stages of pregnancy. Use Lavender with caution if you have low blood pressure.

LEMON

Effects: refreshing, stimulating

Aroma: top note

Scent: fresh, sharp citrus

Combines well with: chamomile, lavender, ylang ylang

Properties: antiseptic, astringent, antiviral, stimulant

Uses: cellulite, chilblains, circulatory problems, cold Sores, constipation, corns, gingivitis, headaches, insect bites, migraine, rheumatism, sinusitis, skin tonic, sore throat, tonsillitis, varicose veins

Contra-indications: Lemon is a photosensitizer (increases the skins reaction to sunlight making it more likely to burn) so it should not be used when exposed to sunlight or tanning beds. Lemon should not be directly inhaled.

LEMONGRASS

Effects: refreshing, toning

Aroma: top note

Scent: sweet, citrus

Combines well with: basil, cedarwood, lavender

Properties: antidepressant, antiseptic, diuretic

Uses: colic, fatigue, indigestion, muscle aches and pains, stimulates appetite, stress

Contra-indications: None known.

MARJORAM

Effects: soothing, warming

Aroma: middle note
Scent: warm, spicy
Combines well with: bergamot, cedarwood, lavender
Properties: analgesic, antiseptic, Antispasmodic, diuretic
Uses: anxiety, arthritis, bronchitis, bruises, colic, constipation, digestive problems, flatulence, insomnia, muscle aches and pains, PMS symptoms, rheumatism, sinusitis, sprains
Contra-indications: Marjoram has antispasmodic properties so use during pregnancy not advised.

MELISSA/LEMON BALM
Effects: uplifting, refreshing
Aroma: middle note
Scent: fresh, sweet, herbal
Combines well with: bergamot, eucalyptus, geranium
Properties: antidepressant, antispasmodic, sedative
Uses: acne, cold sores, colds, cough, flu, PMS symptoms, stress
Contra-indications: Melissa/lemon balm may cause skin irritation. Use well diluted. Do not use during pregnancy.

MYRRH
Effects: toning, rejuvenating
Aroma: middle note
Scent: warm, spicy (similar to musk)
Combines well with: clove, frankincense, geranium
Properties: analgesic, antiseptic, astringent, expectorant
Uses: arthritis, bronchitis, colds, cough, digestive problems, mouth and gum problems, stimulates immune system
Contra-indications: Myrrh should not be used during pregnancy.

NEROLI
Effects: relaxing
Aroma: top note
Scent: floral, refreshing
Combines well with: chamomile, lavender, sandalwood

Properties: antidepressant, antiseptic, antispasmodic, sedative
Uses: depression, digestive problems, dry or sensitive skin,
    flatulence, headaches, insomnia, irritable bowel syndrome,
    nervous tension, panic attacks, stress
Contra-indications: Neroli has antispasmodic properties and
    should not be used during pregnancy.

ORANGE
Effects: refreshing, relaxing
Aroma: top note
Scent: fresh, citrus
Combines well with: frankincense, lavender, rosemary
Properties: antidepressant, antiseptic, antispasmodic,
    detoxifying, sedative, tonic
Uses: anxiety, cellulite, constipation, depression, diarrhea,
    digestive problems, dry, sensitive, or aging skin, flatulence,
    indigestion, insomnia, muscle aches and pains, nervous
    tension, respiratory conditions, stress
Contra-indications: Orange has antispasmodic properties
    and should not be used during pregnancy. Orange may
    irritate sensitive skin (use well diluted). Orange is also a
    photosensitizer (increases the skin's reaction to sunlight
    making it more likely to burn) so it should not be used when
    exposed to sunlight or tanning beds.

PATCHOULI
Effects: relaxing
Aroma: base note
Scent: sweet, spicy, woody
Combines well with: geranium, lavender, neroli
Properties: antidepressant, anti-inflammatory, antiseptic,
    astringent, diuretic, sedative
Uses: anxiety, cellulite, chapped/cracked skin, depression,
    eczema, increase libido, PMS symptoms, scar tissue, water
    retention
Contra-indications: None known.

PEPPERMINT
Effects: refreshing, stimulating
Aroma: top note
Scent: strong, fresh, menthol
Combines well with: eucalyptus, lavender, rosemary
Properties: analgesic, antiseptic, antispasmodic, astringent, decongestant, digestive aid, expectorant
Uses: asthma, bronchitis, colic, headaches, indigestion, insect repellant, migraine, muscle and joint pain, nausea, sinusitis, sore/tired feet, toothaches
Contra-indications: Peppermint has antispasmodic properties therefore use during pregnancy is not advised.

PETITGRAIN
Effects: restoring, stimulating
Aroma: top note
Scent: sweet, floral, woody
Combines well with: bergamot, lavender, other citrus oils
Properties: antibacterial, antidepressant, anti-fungal, antiseptic, antispasmodic, stimulant
Uses: acne, anxiety, digestive problems, exhaustion, insomnia, respiratory problems, stress
Contra-indications: Petitgrain has antispasmodic properties therefore use during pregnancy is not advised.

PINE
Effects: refreshing, stimulating
Aroma: middle note
Scent: fresh, woody
Combines well with: eucalyptus, geranium, lavender
Properties: antiseptic, decongestant, disinfectant, expectorant, tonic
Uses: bronchitis, cystitis, disinfectant, flu, gout, laryngitis, muscle aches and pains, respiratory problems, rheumatism, sinusitis
Contra-indications: Pine may cause skin irritation in sensitive skin.

ROSE
Effects: relaxing
Aroma: base/middle note
Scent: warm, deep floral
Combines well with: bergamot, chamomile, geranium
Properties: antibacterial, antidepressant, antiseptic,
    antispasmodic, astringent, diuretic, sedative
Uses: aging skin, broken veins, depression, dry skin, headache,
    insomnia, PMS symptoms, sensitive skin, sore throat, stress
Contra-indications: Rose has antispasmodic properties and
    should not be used during pregnancy.

ROSEMARY
Effects: refreshing, stimulating
Aroma: middle note
Scent: refreshing, woody, herbal
Combines well with: cedarwood, geranium, juniper
Properties: analgesic, antidepressant, anti-rheumatic, antiseptic,
    antispasmodic, decongestant, diuretic, stimulant
Uses: burns, cellulite, colds, digestive problems, fatigue, flu,
    gout, liver and gall
bladder problems, oily skin, poor circulation, rheumatism,
    water retention, wounds
Contra-indications: Rosemary has antispasmodic properties
    and should not be used during pregnancy or if you have high
    blood pressure or epilepsy.

SANDALWOOD
Effects: warming, relaxing
Aroma: base note
Scent: woody, sweet, exotic
Combines well with: frankincense, geranium, jasmine
Properties: anti-inflammatory, antiseptic, antispasmodic,
    aphrodisiac, diuretic, sedative
Uses: anxiety, bronchitis, cystitis, fatigue, frigidity, impotence,
    immune system booster, nervous tension, skin conditions

(such as acne, dry skin, eczema), sore throat, stress, urinary infections, water retention

Contra-indications: Sandalwood has antispasmodic properties and should not be used during pregnancy or in states of depression (may cause an even lowered mood).

TEA TREE
Effects: cleansing, refreshing
Aroma: top note
Scent: fresh, medicinal
Combines well with: Best used on its own
Properties: antibiotic, anti-fungal, antiseptic, antiviral, detoxifying, insecticide, stimulant
Uses: age spots, athlete's foot, boils, burns, catarrh, colds, corns, cystitis, dandruff, fungal infections, immune system booster, itching (from insect bites, chicken pox, etc.), sunburn, urinary tract infections, warts
Contra-indications: Tea tree has antispasmodic properties and should not be used during pregnancy or if you have high blood pressure. Avoid prolonged use, as toxicity is possible.

THYME
Effects: refreshing, warming
Aroma: top note
Scent: sweet, strong, herbal
Combines well with: bergamot, cedarwood, chamomile
Properties: anti-rheumatic, antiseptic, antispasmodic, aphrodisiac, diuretic, emmenagogue, expectorant
Uses: arthritis, colds, cough, depression, immune system booster, fatigue, laryngitis, memory (enhances), raises low blood pressure, rheumatism, sore throat, stress, tonsillitis
Contra-indications: Thyme may irritate sensitive skin.

VETIVER
Effects: relaxing
Aroma: base note

Scent: heavy, woody, earthy
Combines well with: geranium, lavender, rose
Properties: antibacterial, anti-fungal, antiseptic, sedative
Uses: arthritis, cleanses the aura (energy field around the body)
   to keep out disease, exhaustion, insomnia, nervousness, skin
   disorders (acne, aging skin), stress
Contra-indications: None known.

YLANG YLANG
Effects: relaxing, stimulating
Aroma: base/middle note
Scent: heavy, sweet, floral, exotic
Combines well with: cedarwood, clary sage, geranium
Properties: antidepressant, antiseptic, aphrodisiac, sedative
Uses: anxiety, high blood pressure, intestinal problems, sexual
   dysfunction, stress
Contra-indications: Ylang ylang may irritate sensitive skin. Do
   not use on inflammatory skin conditions and dermatitis.
   Ylang ylang has a strong aroma and may cause headaches.

Appendix 4
Reiki

The simple path to health and happiness

Nowadays many people have heard of Reiki. It is becoming as well known as other mainstream complementary therapies like reflexology and aromatherapy. When you hear about Reiki for the first time you might think, "Oh no, not another New-Age therapy," but really Reiki is more of an "old age" therapy! It has been around in one form or another since "beginning-less" time. It is a very ancient, tried, and tested path to health and happiness.

Dr. Mikao Usui was the founder of Reiki in its present form; he was a Buddhist monk living in Japan in the last century. Dr. Usui had a keen interest in the healing arts and sciences and he had a great passion to relieve the suffering of others, especially the sick. It was this drive, coupled with his understanding of the body and mind, that led him on a fascinating journey to discover a simple method of healing that anyone could practice successfully. This he achieved and you can read about his fascinating quest in many of the books on Reiki that are now available.

So, what is Reiki? Well, on one level we can say that it is a very simple hands-on healing technique for body and mind. In fact, it is so simple that it is literally "Hands On – Reiki On," "Hands Off – Reiki Off"! When a Reiki practitioner places her or his hands on or near the patient there begins an immediate flow or transfer of "healing energy." This is a wonderful thing to experience, very peaceful, very calming, and very natural. During a full Reiki treatment the practitioner will place their hands in about 12 different positions on or near the front and back of the body and this might last up to an hour.

This healing energy is Reiki or Universal Life Force Energy as it is translated from Japanese. It could also be called Universal Chi or Qi. Many of us have heard about Chi or Qi. We know that many of the Eastern philosophies and healing systems talk about it and that it exists in many forms. Subtle life force energy (chi/qi) runs through invisible pathways or meridians in the human body and when these are blocked or imbalanced, due to stress for example, then illness and increased stress can result. Many complementary therapies like acupuncture are based on an intimate knowledge of the human energy system. Our thoughts and emotions also "ride" on subtle internal energy so if we are carrying poor quality internal energy it is easy for us to become "down" and negative and in turn this can encourage the downward spiral to poor health.

Different types or levels or frequencies of life force energy exist in all living things like animals, plants, trees, rocks, and crystals. Life force energy is the basic force of life – it makes plants grow, planets turn, birds sing, and so on – without it nothing would exist. There is an abundance of this pure energy in the countryside or by the sea. But in built-up areas this natural life-giver is often restricted or of poor quality. However, there are many ways we can combat this. Apart from giving and receiving Reiki one way is to regularly and consistently think positively and compassionately and practice contentment. This naturally improves our internal chi and wards off ill-health and unhappiness. A good way to develop these qualities is to learn some simple meditation techniques.

Essentially Reiki is a very pure form of subtle energy and when it is introduced to the body it naturally removes or "transmutes" subtle energy blockages and purifies or raises the quality of our own internal energies. The immediate effects of this are often more energy, feeling more relaxed, and being more able to deal with the daily hassles of life with a positive mind. But there is also often a feeling of coming home to yourself and becoming more aware that you are much more than just a physical and mental being. The presence of Reiki serves to reconnect us to our divinity, our true nature. It can bring us to a fresh awareness of ourselves and help us see our lives and the world around us in a new light. These changes can be very subtle and it is often others who point them out and say things like, "you seem different" or "you seem more relaxed and at peace"! There is definitely a sense of increased contentment and peace of mind with those who practice or receive Reiki.

The great beauty of Reiki is that anyone can become a Reiki practitioner in a matter of days. All we need to do is find a Reiki teacher with whom we feel comfortable and then take the First Degree course. This will teach you how to treat yourself and others. The main focal point of the course is the attunements or empowerments that begin, open, and expand your capacity to channel Reiki. This is a wonderful experience for many people and is often the beginning of a lifelong journey toward good health and personal happiness.

There are many accounts of how effective Reiki has been in combating illness and improving the quality of lives. People from all walks of life and from all cultures and religions practice Reiki. Many people interpret or explain Reiki based on their own religious beliefs, Christians may say that it is a manifestation of the Holy Spirit, Buddhists might say that it is Buddha's blessings, and so on. Reiki is a very experiential phenomenon: it is difficult to describe, define or categorize the true essence of Reiki.

There is no doubt that in this new millennium we are encountering many changes in society and the way we experience and understand life. There are many new opportunities and we have to be open enough not to miss the boat but critical enough to separate the gold from the dross. You can use Reiki as a simple but very effective healing technique, but in the greater context Reiki also gives us the opportunity to broaden your internal horizons, expand your spiritual awareness, and finally find some true peace of mind, if that is what you wish.

Why learn Reiki?

Reiki is a well-known and respected, simple yet profound system of hands-on healing that transcends cultural and religious boundaries. It is also a gentle yet powerful path to personal and spiritual growth. Reiki can have a profound effect on health and well-being by rebalancing, cleansing, and renewing our subtle internal energy system. Here are a few examples of the many ways you can use Reiki as a "hands-on" healing technique, or by simply setting mental intentions:

- To heal yourself and others physically, mentally and emotionally
- For personal growth, healing deep-seated personal issues and developing compassion, empathy, wisdom, patience, and other good qualities
- To heal animals and plants
- To heal relationship problems at work or home
- To send healing energy to world situations such as wars and natural disasters, or local situations such as crime, unemployment and poverty
- To complement and strengthen other therapies such as aromatherapy, reflexology, counseling etc.
- To find new employment, a new house, car, or anything else!
- To have a safe and swift journey while traveling
- To find a solution to a specific problem
- To calm yourself before going into stressful situations such as exams, interviews, or public speaking
- To always be blessed, guided, and protected

There are so many ways we can use Reiki, the only limitations are our imagination and faith. By developing the courage to let go and experience the true essence of Reiki we can begin to realize our true nature as a whole and healthy physical, mental, and spiritual being. Learning Reiki can become the first step on a very enjoyable and enlightening journey toward realizing our true potential, whatever we perceive that to be.

There are many fascinating aspects to Reiki. If you want to know more read *Reiki for Beginners* (Llewellyn) or *Reiki Mastery* (O Books) by David Vennells or contact one of the following organizations:

THE REIKI ALLIANCE
PO Box 41,
Cataldo,
ID83810,
USA.
Tel: 1 208 682 3535.
Fax: 1 208 682 4848.
E-mail: 75051.3471@compuserve.com

THE REIKI ALLIANCE
Cornbrook Bridge House,
Clee Hill,
Ludlow,
Shropshire,
SY8 3QQ,
UK
Tel/fax: 01584 891197.
E-mail: KateReikiJones@compuserve.com

UK REIKI FEDERATION
PO Box 1785,
Andover,
Hampshire.
Tel: 01264 773774.
E-mail: enquiry@reikifed.co.uk
www.reikifed.co.uk

Appendix 5

The metamorphic technique

The following information is kindly provided by the Metamorphic Association, www.metamorphicassociation. org.uk.

What does a session of the Metamorphic Technique involve?

A session usually lasts for about an hour. The recipient removes their shoes and socks and may be either sitting or lying down. The practitioner uses a light touch on the spinal reflex points in the feet, hands, and head. Sessions are non-diagnostic: the practitioner does not seek to address specific symptoms or problems, so there is no need to take a case history. Some people may wish to talk about it and that is fine, but it is not necessary.

Metamorphic Technique practitioners work in a detached way. This does not mean that they don't care. It simply means that they do not make judgments, impose their will, or seek to direct the other person's life force in any way. This creates an environment in which that person's life force is free to do whatever is needed. The person is empowered to be his or her own healer. Most people find sessions very pleasant and relaxing.

Is the Metamorphic Technique a therapy?

The Metamorphic Technique is not a therapy or a treatment, as it is not concerned with addressing specific symptoms or problems. There is no need for practitioners to know about your personal or medical history. The technique is gentle, non-invasive, and completely safe. It can be used on its own or alongside conventional medicine or alternative and complementary therapies. It is easy to learn and, since no special abilities or background are needed, it is accessible to everyone.

Whereas people may seek medicine or therapy because they want to be healed of something, they come to the Metamorphic Technique because they want to transform their patterns. It is an empowering tool for enabling people to "get out of their own way," let go of past limitations, and move forward in their lives.

What happens after a session?

Practitioners cannot predict or guarantee what will happen after a session because this depends on each person's own life force, which is unique. People often feel energized or relaxed, or both. As their energy shifts, people may sometimes re-experience some past symptoms or some emotional upset over a day or two. This is all part of the process of bringing up old patterns to be released. Thankfully, while the life force can bring about great shifts, they always seem to be at a level that people can cope with.

In some cases changes are immediately noticeable, while in others they are more subtle. These changes can range from significant improvements in physical, mental, or emotional health to general feelings of having more energy and confidence, releasing old habits, or gradually letting go of past hurts. People often report significant changes in the way they see life and how they feel about themselves; in many cases they experience a growing sense of purpose and inner strength and may find themselves changing their job, moving house, leaving a relationship, or finding a new one as their life "gets on track." Some people have described it as being like "coming home to themselves."

One thing that is noticed time and again as people receive sessions, is that they change for the better.

How many sessions are needed and how often?

It is entirely up to each person to determine the number and frequency of sessions received. Some people have regular weekly sessions, while others have sessions every so often or when they feel the need. As everyone is different, practitioners cannot predict how long it will take for changes to happen. Sometimes people begin to notice changes after just one session; for others it may take weeks or even months. Each person's life force will bring about changes in whatever timescale is right for them. While changes may not always be immediate, they do tend to be permanent.

Is the Metamorphic Technique suitable for everyone?

Yes. The Metamorphic Technique is gentle, non-invasive, and completely safe. As it is the person's own life force that does the healing, it cannot do any harm. It can be safely used by anyone including children, pregnant mothers, and people who are dying.
The technique can be received on its own or alongside other approaches, whether conventional medicine or alternative and complementary therapies.

What can the Metamorphic Technique do for me?

As the name suggests, the Metamorphic Technique is concerned with change and transformation, which can occur on a number of levels – physical, mental, emotional, and behavioral.

While practitioners cannot predict the outcome, as each person's life force is unique, the majority of people who have experienced the technique do report benefits – it is unusual for the technique not to be helpful in some way.

People are often drawn to the Metamorphic Technique at difficult times such as illness, bereavement, divorce, and so on, or because they feel at a crossroads or "stuck" in their lives. They find that it can help them to cope better in these difficult or transitional times.

Many people are drawn to the technique because it allows them to deal with emotional issues and make deep inner changes without having to discuss their problems or delve into their past. On a physical level, people come with a variety of conditions from cancer to chronic fatigue. The Technique does not seek to address these conditions or their symptoms; however, in many cases people find that symptoms diminish over time, or that they respond better to other treatments they have been following.

The Metamorphic Technique has been used a great deal in work with physical and mental disabilities, as well as in schools for children with learning difficulties, in hospitals, in prisons, and in helping people overcome addictions, eating disorders, and stress-related conditions. It is also used by pregnant women and midwives, as it can allow an easier pregnancy and birth. Above all, the Metamorphic Technique is suitable for anyone who wishes to make changes that will enhance their quality of life.

Can anyone learn the Metamorphic Technique?

Yes. Although the theory behind it can initially seem quite difficult to grasp, the practice is very simple to learn and use. No special abilities or background are needed to practice. It does not involve diagnosis, so no medical training is needed. Many people take short courses so they can use the Technique with family and friends. Parents are especially encouraged to learn, so they can give the Technique to their children.

How was it developed?

The Metamorphic Technique has its origins in the work of Robert St. John, a British naturopath and reflexologist. During the 1960s he discovered that he could bring about significant changes by applying a light touch to particular points on the feet that reflexologists call the spinal reflexes. Later, he realized that everyone has their own capacity for self-healing and that, if he allowed it to become fully active while practicing, then his patients would be empowered to be their own healers in a truly effective way. Since permanent, far-reaching changes on a number of levels were now occurring in his patients – changes originating entirely from within the patients themselves – he developed a body of work aptly named Metamorphosis. This unique approach distinguished it from the temporary, limited changes that his previous therapeutic approaches had achieved.

Gaston Saint-Pierre, who studied extensively with Robert St. John during the 1970s, saw the potential for the development of a practical tool for self-healing and the realization of one's potential that could be easily integrated into everyday life. He therefore went on to further develop the work and created the term "The Metamorphic Technique" to differentiate the new direction the work was now taking. The word "technique" is defined as a way of approaching a task that perfects itself in the practice. In 1979 he set up the Metamorphic Association, which was then registered as a charity in 1984, to promote the Technique worldwide.

What is the theory behind the Metamorphic Technique?

From the traditions of Eastern medicine to the new discoveries of science, it is generally acknowledged that energy or "life force" underlies all forms of life. This is the basis for the Metamorphic Technique. It is now widely recognized that our energy can get "stuck" in particular patterns. Every cell that makes up our bodies and minds holds memories of our experiences – not only from our childhood but going right back through our time in the womb to the moment we were conceived. When an experience affects us strongly, the thoughts, emotions, and beliefs connected to that memory can set up energy patterns in which we become "stuck." In a sense, they keep us stuck in the past. These energy patterns can express themselves in a variety of ways, such as physical or mental illness, emotional problems, limiting attitudes and beliefs, or repeating patterns of behavior. In fact, the Metamorphic Technique sees all mental, emotional, physical, and behavioral "problems" as symptoms or expressions of energy patterns.

By using a light touch to the spinal reflex points on the feet, hands, and head, the Metamorphic practitioner acts as a catalyst (something that speeds up a process of change) to the person's life force. The life force, guided by the person's innate intelligence, will then bring about whatever transformations of the energy patterns are needed. This enables the person to naturally shift those patterns that no longer serve them. The energy that was "stuck" is released, freeing them up from past influences and allowing them to let go and move forward. While the theory can initially seem quite difficult to grasp, it is not necessary to understand it to benefit.

What is unique about the Metamorphic Technique?

The Metamorphic Technique is:

- A unique tool for personal transformation.
- Not a therapy or a treatment, but a technique that helps trigger your own inner life force, enabling you to better realize your potential.

- Based on a new way of looking at energy patterns. While other approaches often focus on removing energy blockages, the Metamorphic Technique looks at transforming energy patterns. It does not consider people to be "blocked" or "broken" and in need of being "fixed." Instead, it simply notices that you may have patterns that no longer serve you and that you wish to transform. The energy that was involved in creating the old patterns is released and can be used to create new patterns.
- Empowering. Any changes that occur originate entirely from within the recipient. That person's own life force has an innate intelligence of its own. The practitioner simply acts as a catalyst in the process.
- Non-invasive. There is no physical manipulation, no diagnosis, and no need to discuss personal problems or medical history.
- Gentle and completely safe.
- Accessible to everyone, and easy to learn and integrate into everyday life.

Appendix 6
Bach flower remedies

The Bach remedies represent the highest, most positive and altruistic of human qualities and although they were originally conceived as remedies to cure illness they can also be used to help us develop whatever positive qualities we may be lacking. In fact the Bach remedies can be a great support to the process of spiritual development and personal growth. If we believe that all illness has its root in the mind, as Dr. Bach did, we could also say that using the remedies is a form of preventative medicine. In fact we can regard all our positive thoughts, words, and deeds as preventative medicine!

The remedies can help us develop our positive qualities and abandon negative attitudes. In the short run positive thoughts and emotions create a sense of contentment and well-being and in the long run, if we believe that what we "put out" into the world eventually comes back to us, then we are also investing in a healthy and happy future.

Through his early study and research Dr. Bach became aware that to find a truly effective form of healing that would strike at the root of ill-health he would have to understand the true causes of illness. This led him in a similar direction to Samuel Hahnemann, the founder of homeopathy, and to the idea that the true cause and cure of disease is not simply a physical phenomenon but mental in origin. The physical symptoms of disease are simply an external manifestation of inner dis-ease. Despite the fact that they both had little knowledge of psychology they were still able to deduce that successful remedies would have to work on the mental origins of the malady to effect a lasting cure.

Dr. Bach knew that he would have to discover remedies that would work on the subtle mental and emotional levels of the mind; he would have to find remedies that were able to dispel negative states of mind and promote positive ones. These remedies would have to be specific enough to target the particular negative states of mind that were giving rise to the physical symptoms. He must have realized from homeopathy that the patient's state of mind could be improved when the appropriate remedy was prescribed and this would give rise to good physical health. He must have also realized that the homeopathic remedy carried some form of healing energy or life force that directly improved the patient's frame of mind and physical health.

Bach and Hahnemann were men of great wisdom and their discoveries and philosophies were way ahead of their time and still way ahead of modern psychology and medicine. Both their systems of medicine have achieved incredible results and have brought great benefit to countless people.

Dr. Bach wanted his remedies to be so simple to use that anyone could select and take them without professional advice or the need for any special techniques. That is why the simple method set out here is still the only one used by the Bach Centre and by the practitioners on its register.

Imagine, for example, that you are suffering from asthma. There is no Bach Flower Remedy for asthma, since this is a physical complaint. Instead you need to ignore the asthma and look at the kind of person you are. Perhaps you are someone who is shy and timid, and who gets nervous about things like speaking in public and meeting new people. This would indicate that you are a *mimulus* type, so this would be the first remedy to select.

Then you might think about the way you are feeling at the moment. Perhaps your son is about to start school and quite without cause you are frightened that he will be bullied. *Red chestnut* is the remedy for the fear that something bad will happen to loved ones. Perhaps you have been working too hard and are exhausted: this would indicate the need for *olive*.

You can select up to six or seven different remedies in this way. Don't worry too much if you make a wrong selection, because if a remedy is not needed it will not do anything. Experience has shown, however, that too many remedies taken at one time are not as effective as a few well-chosen ones. This means that there is no point mixing all 38 together to zap everything at once!

Each of the 38 remedies discovered by Dr. Bach is directed at a particular characteristic or emotional state. To select the remedies you need you only need to think about the sort of person you are and the way you are feeling. Then you take the remedies you need.

Here is a list of the 38 remedies with brief indications:

Agrimony – mental torture behind a cheerful face
Aspen – fear of unknown things
Beech – intolerance
Centaury – the inability to say "no"
Cerato – lack of trust in one's own decisions
Cherry plum – fear of the mind giving way
Chestnut bud – failure to learn from mistakes
Chicory – selfish, possessive love
Clematis – dreaming of the future without working in the present
Crab apple – the cleansing remedy, also for self-hatred
Elm – overwhelmed by responsibility
Gentian – discouragement after a setback
Gorse – hopelessness and despair
Heather – self-centeredness and self-concern
Holly – hatred, envy, and jealousy
Honeysuckle – living in the past
Hornbeam – procrastination, tiredness at the thought of doing something
Impatiens – impatience
Larch – lack of confidence

Mimulus – fear of known things

Mustard – deep gloom for no reason

Oak – the plodder who keeps going past the point of
    exhaustion

Olive – exhaustion following mental or physical effort

Pine – guilt

Red chestnut – over-concern for the welfare of loved ones

Rock rose – terror and fright

Rock water – self-denial, rigidity and self-repression

Scleranthus – inability to choose between alternatives

Star of Bethlehem – shock

Sweet chestnut – Extreme mental anguish, when everything
    has been tried and there is no light left

Vervain – over-enthusiasm

Vine – dominance and inflexibility

Walnut – protection from change and unwanted influences

Water violet – pride and aloofness

White chestnut – unwanted thoughts and mental
    arguments

Wild oat – uncertainty over one's direction in life

Wild rose – drifting, resignation, apathy

Willow – self-pity and resentment

You can take the remedies in several ways. For the treatment of a short-term mood or problem the easiest way is to put two drops of each selected remedy in a glass of water and sip as required, but at least four times a day, until relief is obtained. If using Rescue Remedy, put in four drops instead of two. For the treatment of more chronic problems you should make up a treatment bottle, as this is more economical and will make the precious stock remedies go a bit further. Simply get a 30ml bottle with a dropper in the lid (try the local pharmacy), and then add two drops of each selected remedy (four drops of Rescue Remedy) to the bottle. Top this up with still mineral water and from this bottle take four drops four times a day.

If you keep them in the fridge, treatment bottles will last from two to four weeks. If you can't keep your bottle in the fridge but have to keep it in your pocket or handbag then you can add a teaspoon of brandy to the treatment bottle – this will help to keep the water from going off. If you don't want to use brandy, cider vinegar is an alternative, although it isn't quite so effective.

For more information on the Bach Flower Remedies visit www.bachflowercentre.com or read *Bach Flower Remedies for Beginners* by David Vennells (published by Llewellyn).

Index